Stronger Than Sickness

Staying Empowered Through Illness

Rochelle Bohannon

ISBN-13: 978-1543202526
ISBN-10: 1543202527

Dedication

To my mama: Thank you for taking care of me while we walked this incredible journey together. I couldn't have done any of it without you.

To my husband: You are the best choice that I have ever made. Thank you for insisting that this book come to life and pushing me harder than ever to own my voice and inspire others.

Table of Contents

Introduction

Health isn't the absence of sickness. Sickness is the absence of health.

You are likely reading this book because you are suffering from a debilitating illness and struggling to navigate the dark, crazy waters that come along with it. That, or you are in a close relationship with someone who has experienced the unparalleled frustration in existing as a sort of medical anomaly.

I am here to tell you one very important thing:

Your frustration is your fuel.

We all know someone who is sick. I'm not talking about a benign virus or even something more identifiably serious. I'm talking about symptoms that come virtually out of nowhere and have no definitive cause; symptoms that completely uproot the possibility of living life comfortably. We can probably all think of someone that we know (or a friend of a friend) who has experienced a health crisis of some kind.

Human beings are living longer than ever before, but we are also much sicker than we have ever been. I'm not talking about historically awful diseases like the measles, smallpox, polio, cholera, or the bubonic plague. I'm talking about cancers, chronic sickness, allergies, and reactions that we aren't yet able to understand. So many people become sick and suffer for months or years. They become lost, both physically and emotionally, in a cycle of pain and frustration. It's dark and lonely and something that no one should have to endure.

There are many theories on what the triggers might be but so far, not many answers. Some suspect that genetics play a role. Others point to chemicals and contamination in the environment. Perhaps it's a combination of these factors, an underlying susceptibility that lies dormant until a trigger—environmental or viral—activates the disease.

When your health is in crisis, you feel lost, overwhelmed, disheartened, and probably a little pissed off too. How do I know this? **Because I've been there.** I spent upwards of six years existing as a medical anomaly, totally lost, perpetually frustrated, and in desperate need of empowerment, clarity, guidance and intention.

This book will give you exactly that. *Stronger Than Sickness* will give you a warm sense of direction and empower you as you navigate this crazy and unexpected journey.

During my own six-year health crisis, I felt overwhelmingly alone. I would spend hours upon hours researching various medical conditions with no break in the case. I desperately wanted out. I was unable to act proactively in the entire process, largely because it was so exhausting, overwhelming and a total buzz kill to my optimism.

When you are sick, the uncertainty is frustrating at the least and frightening at the worst. Patients may go months or years without the answers and guidance they need and that typically translates to a complete lack of proper treatment and a downward spiral of their condition. You become further debilitated, either by way of the original illness or at the hands of various side effects via medications or attempts at treatment. Everything surrounding your illness can easily become blurred and oftentimes, the course of treatment now involves treating all of your symptoms rather than the original cause, which creates a cycle that confuses everyone involved. And so begins a long and frustrating fight that over time, seems nearly impossible to endure.

Bottom line: a health crisis can be tremendously disempowering.

So what do you do now?

Now, you acknowledge to yourself that you have the right to live a healthy, happy life. You look for support. You ask for respect as a patient and as a human. You take this challenge and resolve to utilize everything out there to bring yourself back to health. ***Most importantly, you never give up on finding and living your health.***

I wish I had read something like this when I was in the thick of it. It took me a long time to figure out what was going on inside of my body physically, and even longer to process it all mentally and emotionally. I had a multitude of highs and lows that never seemed to yield me any progress and although research became my best friend, I was missing the very thing that I hope this book can bring to those in a similar situation: **a warm, understanding, and inspiring point of reference.**

And now, here I am, very much on the other side of it. I know that it can be tremendously difficult to form clear intentions and take precise action, particularly when it comes to your own well-being, but even more so when you are at the mercy of a raging illness. I walked this path and I know first hand just how lonely that place can feel. **But you are not alone.**

Now, I can't promise a definitive (or ideal) solution here. Trust me, I wish more than anything that my super powers extended into this realm of possibility and that I could run around with healing magic so that no one ever has to experience anything like I did. But everyone's "solution" looks different. Some are impressively clear and others are a jumbled mess (like mine!). Some are definitive and some won't ever be (wholly) solved.

The point is, of course, that you want to solve this. **But this book isn't about your solution; it's about navigating your path to health intentionally.** It's about taking a look at every single aspect of your life in the midst of this chaos. It's about intentionally living your best life in the face of this crisis so that you can live an even better life once you get through it.

What I *can* promise you is this: once you take an intentional approach, your solution will come. I say this with 100% certainty because every single method outlined within these pages is one that has done incredible things for me, both physically and emotionally.

My journey was messy, but this book is meant to bring you some structure. It's your beacon of light, and ultimately it's the beginning of your journey back to health.

Crazy as it might sound, this illness is ultimately your gift. Take control of your life right now by opening it.

My Story

DISCLOSURE: I am fully aware that you are in the throes of your own health crisis and reading my story might the last thing that you feel like doing at the moment. I say this because I would have probably felt the same way. Feel free to skim read this or to skip it entirely. I know that you have your own fight to fight right now and the next few pages might not be of any immediate help to you. Perhaps you will come back to it and perhaps you won't. Either way, I wanted to include it for those who might find a parallel experience helpful, to illustrate how messy and misguided it all was, and to show exactly why I wanted to create something that helps to streamline this process for someone else. Most importantly, it's my street cred on this topic and testimony that I've been there and I came out of it. **It's also proof that you can too.**

My illness manifested very abruptly in the spring of my junior year of high school. I was seventeen and exploring all of those crazy, irrational, and exciting trials that the teenage years typically bring. I felt normal. I looked normal. But one evening, that sense of normalcy was entirely lost.

I had been feeling a little strange all afternoon. I chalked it up to the emotional havoc that a first love can bring and carried on through dinner, but in the middle of our meal I began to feel an unfamiliar abdominal pain. It was sharp, came in waves, and brought with it a ton of nausea. I started to throw up. I quickly drove myself home, continued to vomit for many hours, lost consciousness, and woke up in the emergency room with a tube down my throat. My mom had come home to find me sprawled on the bathroom floor, completely disoriented, and she promptly drove me to the emergency room.

I stayed in the hospital for eight days. During this time, I was unable to eat anything. I was ravenous, but any time I attempted to consume anything except water, it came right back up. You name the test, I had it done. My gastroenterologist was concerned but completely perplexed. I was asked questions that very much insinuated that this was some type of eating disorder. Then they brought in a neurologist to examine a small benign cyst that showed up on my brain in a CT scan (these are apparently totally normal, but as you can imagine, shook us up quite a bit). The neurologist mentioned that I was displaying potential symptoms of "abdominal migraines" but offered a very vague explanation of what this could really mean.

And there was one more thing: my doctor reviewed my blood work and noted that my amylase and lipase levels were ever so slightly elevated at the time that I was admitted to the hospital. I remember him saying that this might be indicative of pancreatitis but typically, these levels would be astronomically higher than normal. In my case, they were more on the "high-end" of normal.

The non-stop research began right here, with pancreatitis and abdominal migraines.

I left the hospital and went to prom a few days later. I carried on. I continued to have similar attacks for months, although they didn't always manifest in the exact same way. Sometimes they lasted for two days and sometimes it was longer. Every time, though, the pain was the same. It was utterly debilitating and the only relief that could be found was in a trip to the emergency room and a nice dose of Dilaudid for the pain and Phenergan for the nausea. Typically, after this, my body would calm down, snap out of it, and a few days later I would return to life as "normal."

Of course, when you go into the ER and mention that you have a mysterious illness that needs to be treated with a hardcore narcotic, people become suspicious of you. In hindsight, I totally get it. But in those moments, when the pain was persistent, my vision was blurry from its violence, and I had been heaving for hours on end, the rolling eyes and the skepticism were almost hurtful.

About four months after my first attack, my doctors decided that there might be a chance that my gallbladder was the culprit. It seemed like the most obvious possibility and even though scans showed that on the surface it looked relatively healthy, they insisted that I could still have gallstones that were messing me up.

So I had my gallbladder removed with blind hope that it would cure me. **It didn't.** In addition to the painful recovery, I had another attack within a month. I had one of my organs removed for nothing. At the time, the desperation took over; I blocked out the devastation, and carried on with a nice little scar and no gallbladder.

I graduated high school and entered college with hope. I hoped that I could somehow leave my illness at home and start fresh in a place where no one would see me as "the girl with that weird sickness who may or may not be making it all up." That lasted all of about a month before I was in the Emergency Room with those same persistent symptoms.

In the spirit of full, transparent disclosure, I totally partied my way through college. This was absolutely the worst way to handle my personal life and physical health while battling this confusing illness, but in hindsight, it was my way of coping with the frustration. My "normal" college friends drank and partied so I insisted that I could too. I drank alcohol and ate bad food and tortured my body's circadian rhythm and lived in denial that I was "sick" or "different" than anyone else.

We moved back and forth between pancreatitis, abdominal migraines, and (a new one!) cyclic vomiting syndrome as potential diagnoses. I say "we" because at the time, my mom was my biggest advocate. She and I were like a two-man research team in this process with a totally badass motto: *Never Give Up.* So we didn't. I saw a psychiatrist, a nutritionist, a neurologist, and multiple gastroenterologists. They all offered a confused perspective on my situation but the chaos of my illness made it so hard for my mom and I to receive their input in a way that could be constructive.

It was at this point that I entered into what I like to call the home stretch of the darkness. This was absolutely the darkest hour of my illness. By this time, the emotional and physical fatigue had taken a toll and I was on autopilot. Fueled by a nice cocktail of drugs, bad food, and denial, I meandered my way through this time sloppily and with a very limited sense of purpose. My body felt abused and my mind felt foggy. I developed a pretty intense fear of food despite wanting so badly to be able to sit down and eat without anxiety. I honestly felt like my body was rejecting life.

My trips to the Emergency Room had become a complete ordeal beyond the routine doctor skepticism. I had been poked and prodded to such an extent that my veins had become riddled with scar tissue. It became nearly impossible to get an IV into a vein so that I could receive the medication that I needed for relief. During one visit, I was poked twenty-two times before the nurses were finally able to get a small, fragile IV to stay put in my foot. During another visit, they had to resort to a vein in my neck. It was an agonizing and anxiety-ridden process, knowing how many times and how long it would take in order to stop the pain and feel relief.

Because of this, I was referred by a doctor to have a port placed semi-permanently into my chest in order to ensure easy access to my veins. A port is a small bubble-like apparatus installed beneath the skin with a catheter attached to it that is placed inside of a vein. It is "accessed" through the bubble with a special needle and the idea is that drugs can be administered and blood can be drawn, typically with less discomfort than a traditional IV or needle-stick.

Ports are typically only used in hematology and oncology patients (read: hardcore cases) and even though having it brought so much relief and credibility to my Emergency Room visits, I remember thinking that this was such a heavy addition to my case. On one hand, I was relieved because it took away so much of the everyday anxiety that I faced with my episodes. But on the other hand, it filled me with very somber feelings about my future. I remember looking down and touching it several times a day, wincing at what it stood for and wondering if I would have to live with it forever.

In 2011, my mom found a very knowledgeable GI doctor in Milwaukee who specialized in cyclic vomiting syndrome. We were desperate, so we flew out to see her. She evaluated me and came to many of the same conclusions that so many specialists had half-heartedly suggested to me before: mine was a totally mysterious situation and stress and/or diet may or may not be playing a role in what was going on. But then she pointed us in a direction that would ultimately offer our first glimpse of tangible hope. She suggested that we look into sphincter of Oddi dysfunction. Basically, the sphincter of Oddi is a tiny little muscle that regulates the flow of bile and pancreatic juices that help with digestion. In sphincter of Oddi dysfunction, the sphincter muscle does not open when it should, causing severe abdominal pain.

The funny thing is, we had *very* briefly considered sphincter of Oddi dysfunction before. About two months after my first attack, I saw a doctor in Los Angeles who specialized in all things pancreas related and he did a small procedure with a scope to go down into my digestive tract to see if my sphincter of Oddi was blocked. At that time, it wasn't, but I also wasn't in one of my "attacks."

The fact that this doctor brought it up again initially made me shrug my shoulders, but she explained that since I wasn't in an attack at the time there was still a possibility that my sphincter of Oddi was the culprit here and the ultimate root cause of my illness. She advised me to seek out a doctor locally to do the procedure once more and this time, place a stent into my sphincter of Oddi to keep it open, should another attack occur. We found a local specialist with a solid reputation, scheduled the procedure, and went for it.

Over the next six months or so, I definitely did not experience the miracle 100% cure that I was hoping for, BUT my attacks did become much fewer and further between (I think it was 2-3 attacks in this entire time span, which was a huge improvement from the 2-3 per month that had become the norm). Because there was *some* improvement, we decided to move forward and have a sphincterotomy done. Basically, the doctor would make a tiny slice in my Sphincter of Oddi so that it would stay open permanently despite any potential spasms and never close.

Again, for another six months or so after this final procedure, I experienced a very distinct decrease in my attacks. But they weren't gone permanently, which was equal parts confusing and depressing. I felt like the procedure had been pointless and we had acted on our desperation for nothing. At this point, I was also on a fairly consistent dose of pain and anxiety meds, both in the hospital and outside of it, just to maintain a fairly stable existence. So we started to think about this side of things (the meds) and steered our efforts in a direction that explored them as a potential complication.

In short: I went to rehab.

I met with a renowned local doctor and he explained that I probably did have Sphincter of Oddi dysfunction originally. However, (and this is a BIG however. HUGE. MASSIVE. DID I MENTION HUGE?) he revealed to me a very crucial piece of my cluster of a health puzzle that literally made my heart sink and my jaw drop: one of the most prominent side effects of opiates is, in fact, sphincter of Oddi Dysfunction. So basically, **the very medication that I had been repeatedly treated with was initially relieving, but ultimately perpetuating, my illness.**

Mind. Blown.

How could this not have been brought to my attention sooner? It was confusing. No, it was infuriating. I had seen upwards of ten gastroenterologists on this journey and not one had mentioned this as a possibility. Basically, what was happening was that I was being given these drugs and then abruptly stopping them. This high and low approach to dosage essentially shocks your Sphincter of Oddi and causes the problems I was experiencing. Apparently, this side effect was very much proven and yet, had been grossly neglected in terms of awareness in the medical community.

I spent two weeks detoxing in an inpatient facility. They slowly tapered my dosage down and switched me over to the same drug that they use to detox heroin addicts. It sounds pretty hardcore, but I was actually among a very mixed crowd of people. Some fit the profile of true drug addicts and others were in a similar medically induced drug dependence to mine. It was eye-opening and humbling, and I'll never forget the perspective that I gained in my short time there. When I left, I felt clear. I felt liberated and self-aware, and for the first time in six years, I felt like I was able to make plans for my life.

I left the facility not completely drug free. I remained on a very small dosage of a drug called Subutex and the plan was that I would taper this dose down as far as I could before completely going off of it so as not to upset my Sphincter of

Oddi in the process and cause additional attacks that would surely set my progress back.

Long story short: it took me almost a year and a half to fully come off of Subutex. It was the slowest and most annoying process. There were many times that I would get down to what we thought was a small enough dose and then I would go cold-turkey, only to end up in the hospital with another agonizing attack. By the end, I was literally down to a crumb of a pill and experienced a solid four plus weeks of withdrawal symptoms once I was finally able to stop taking this crumb. I was moody, achy, exhausted, my skin was tingling, and I had horrible shivers and sweats.

And then one day, a few months later, I woke up and thought to myself, *I haven't felt all weird and tingly lately. And I haven't had any abdominal pain whatsoever in months.* I had gradually and finally been freed of my mystery illness and I hadn't even been fully aware of it. The transition was that seamless.

It was around this time that I began to make some major changes in my diet and lifestyle (I'll go into those later) and I felt this intense surge of strength and stability take over within my body. It was so empowering and so invigorating and I made a promise to myself to never let go of this newfound zest for life.

For six years I saw specialist after specialist and repeatedly arrived at dead ends. For six years, I was met with eye rolls and suspicion (almost) every time I walked into the ER retching and doubled over in agonizing pain. I saw more GI doctors, neurologists, and psychiatrists than anyone should ever have to see.

In my case, in the moment (translation: six years) of my illness, I genuinely felt lucky. My diagnosis wasn't immediately classified as life threatening or grave by any means. It wasn't typically incapacitating and on the surface, I was able to fake normalcy fairly well. When I did take the time to (attempt) an explanation to those I felt close enough to, I made sure to brighten my eyes with optimism as I smiled and rambled on about how anyone with a definitive diagnosis (such as cancer) was certainly placed in a more unfortunate health crisis than I was.

But the reality of it was that in the long term, if this illness had played out for the remainder of my existence, **it would have absolutely killed me.** I have no doubt that if I had not been able to bring myself physically and emotionally out of this illness, it would have slowly continued to consume my quality of life and at some point, my life would have ended either at the direct hands of this illness or as a side effect of it's chaos.

I could go on and on in disgust and disappointment in how profoundly the medical community had failed me, because the truth is, they did. Big time. But the lesson that I learned in this process is so valuable and so profound that I can't help but feel grateful for the entire thing. All of it.

Once you finish this book, you'll see why.

Phase 1: ACCEPTANCE

"What you deny or ignore, you delay. What you accept and face, you conquer."

— Robert Tew

When most people (including myself at one point) hear the word "acceptance", they think of rolling over and giving up. But giving up is a submissive act, not one of acceptance. Acceptance implies nothing about the future. If we accept something is true in this moment, we can still absolutely work toward changing it. When you allow yourself to accept your illness in this moment, you aren't caving in, but rather you are opening yourself up to see what's on your plate. Here, you can begin to interact with it, to navigate in and around it.

Acceptance simply means the recognition that the moment is as it is. It doesn't void you of hope because hope in no way depends on the denial of symptoms—it is found in the midst of your symptoms and despite your symptoms. **This phase is about recognizing this as your path and walking steadily down it.**

1. Be Here Now

"Be happy in the moment, that's enough. Each moment is all we need, not more."

— Mother Teresa

We live in a very hyper connected and fast-paced world. Because of this, it's easy to lose ourselves on autopilot and cruise through each day mindlessly. Repeat this every day and, in my opinion, you have a pretty lackluster existence. Life is not meant to be lived in this way and yet, so many of us wake up five, ten, twenty, thirty-plus years later and think to ourselves, *'What the hell have I been doing all of this time?'*

You and I, we are not going to be one of those people. Later, you'll thank your illness for this gift of awareness.

I'm in no way an expert on mindfulness. I was, however, pretty well-versed in the art of cruising along and not really paying attention to where I was going or why I was even waking up in the morning. Eventually, I got sick of this because it wasn't working. It wasn't until I was toward the tail end of my illness journey that mindfulness crept into my life. I was no longer experiencing regular attacks and although I was not quite yet stable enough to call myself "healed," I felt a distinct shift in the way that my mind and body were functioning together. This is when my holistic view of health was really starting to gain some traction and mindfulness naturally evolved with that overall mindset. It felt right and it felt real, and for the first time in my life I realized that I had been living completely void of any real intention whatsoever.

Essentially, I wasn't happy and I knew that I could live better. The shift that I have experienced since finding and implementing the concept of mindfulness into my own life has been incredible. Once it established its role in my own process, it began to affect virtually everything that I do and transformed my life in so many ways.

When we live on autopilot and cruise mindlessly through our days, we miss so much. We miss the simple and beautiful things that surround us on the outside and we also miss what our bodies are telling us on the inside. We become stuck in mechanical and conditioned ways of thinking and living, constantly struggling with things that happened in the past or striving for what's coming next, and we forget about the here and the now. ***We become so focused on doing that we stop living.***

All we have is the here and now. As dark of a reality as that might seem, it is a very whole and very raw truth of life. It's a truth so powerful that I physically feel my own body react when I say and hear those words. So many of us don't recognize life from this perspective. We don't acknowledge that tomorrow is never promised to us because it's such a scary and powerful reality. It's easier to deny it and focus on other things than it is to embrace it and use it as the fuel for pursuing your best life.

Once I made a conscious choice to use it as fuel, this reality no longer scared me—it empowered me. It changed how I saw things and it changed the choices that I made, and probably most importantly, it changed how I reacted to things.

To me, mindfulness can best be put into three simple words: **Be. Here. Now.**

It's mostly about stepping up your awareness, turning off autopilot, taking charge of your life, and living intentionally. It's about consciously recognizing thoughts, feelings, actions, bodily sensations, and surroundings. It's about paying attention to the small, seemingly insignificant, moments in life. Moments like your morning sip of coffee, the smile of a loved one, the glory that is sunlight, your daily shower, and on, and on, and on.

As it pertains to your illness, mindfulness is something that can help to calm you and ground you. It can help you focus on the things that truly matter and release things that don't. It can help you to become as in-tune with your body as possible and recognize that even though you might not have as much control as you'd like, you *do* have control of how you react to each day and even in each moment.

When you are sick, there is absolutely an absence. There's an absence of good health, positive energy, social belonging, and sometimes even hope. In this type of situation, mindfulness helps to establish a presence in this absence. Mindfulness can help you to stay positive and present with your life, despite the absence of stable health.

For example, let's talk about frustration. This was an emotion that I felt constantly through my ordeal. It's an uncomfortable and agitating feeling that we all prefer to avoid, and yet it's one that rears up and grabs us often. Instead of internalizing this emotion or lashing out blindly against it (and wasting valuable time and energy), what might happen if you accepted it? What does it take to work with the feeling of frustration, rather than against it? *The answer is mindfulness.*

If you can be mindful with your emotions, you can use them constructively. Feel them, yes, but also observe them. When you do this and take a step back, you can see what's really happening with greater emotional clarity. This allows you to open both your mind and your heart to any emotion so that it can best serve you without taking away from your end goal.

As you embrace this journey, mindfulness can also help you to find the joy in life when you would otherwise feel depleted of optimism. It can help, not necessarily to distract you, but to allow you to see that in your (challenging) world there are good things, too. It can allow you to feel and exist happily, even on days that literally suck the life out of you.

There is much to be explored when it comes to a mindful approach, but I find it best to keep things as simple as possible. I think the brain responds better to smaller "bursts" of mindfulness rather than something that feels unnatural or all consuming. Allow yourself to take baby steps toward mindfulness rather than trying to go all in. If you start to notice the little things, I promise you, a much bigger shift will come.

And let me tell you, mindfulness is not at all about being perfect or present all of the time. It's mostly just about paying better attention, taking the things that you are given, and accepting them as they are. Every moment is a crucial piece of our life-puzzle and if we can try our best to experience them as fully as possible, there are so many great lessons and feelings to be had in their wake.

2. Never Give Up

When I was growing up, my mom drilled into me the very powerful motto: Never Give Up. This motto was a fundamental key to my upbringing and very much responsible for the person that I am today. Because of this, I will pass it fiercely onto my own children in the hope that it will act as a beacon of light for them in difficult times.

I am well aware that little saying can be cliché, even annoyingly so. It is by no means an original concept, but it is something that I have carried with me my entire life, and that right there is what gives it so much power. It is rooted deep inside of my existence and I feel like it runs wild in my blood. I told you—powerful stuff.

There is a reason these kinds of sayings are clichés—they touch on fundamental truths that exist for humanity, truths that guide us, empower us, and ultimately, truths that allow for us to thrive. When you are struggling in a way that affects your health, a way that interferes with your body's ability to exist peacefully, it can be incredibly difficult to remember that this kind of cliché rings true. But in reality, most problems, even when complex, do have a solution.

I use the term "solution" here in a very loose sense and I'll tell you why: the term solution is typically very focused on solving a problem and includes a distinct end point. It took me a long time to realize that a true solution is not a one-size-fits-all concept, nor is it a destination. A solution is a journey. It can mean many things and look very different to everyone.

Over time, I have realized that we as humans tend to create ideal pictures and scenarios in our heads that originate from a positive intention. These idealistic tendencies carry with them a ton of hope, and I think that is a truly beautiful thing. However, the ideal picture that you carry from the beginning of your journey might not be exactly what your body is ultimately capable of. Chances are, the path to a solution will not unfold exactly as you envisioned it, and this is more than okay.

My advice? Stay flexible on this journey. Bend with your illness, but know that it does not have the power to break you. Never give up on your mission to solve your specific case, but know that the solution might come in an unexpected way.

There's a children's fable that I first heard in my mid-twenties, just as I was beginning to see a light at the end of the tunnel in regards to my illness. It goes something like this:

One day, a farmer's donkey fell down into a well. The animal cried for hours as the farmer tried to figure out what to do. Finally, he decided that it wasn't worth it to save the donkey. The animal was old and the well needed to be covered up anyway. He invited all of his neighbors to come over and help him. They all grabbed shovels and began to throw dirt into the well. At first, the donkey was panicked. Then, all of a sudden, he quieted down. A few shovel loads later, the farmer finally looked down the well and was surprised at what was happening. With every shovel of dirt that fell on his back, the donkey would shake it off and take a step up. As everyone continued to shovel dirt on top of him, he continued to shake it off and move up. Eventually, everyone was amazed as the donkey stepped up over the edge of the well and trotted off!

Moral: Life is going to shovel a ton of dirt on you, but you don't have to let it cover you. We can get out of the deepest, darkest holes by choosing to shake off the "dirt" and rise up.

When it comes to things in life that are worth fighting for, your health is at the very top of the list. Good, stable health is the pillar for all that we do in life. Without it, the struggle permeates into all other aspects of how we live, from our relationships to our career and all that lies in between.

I know that there are times in life (even aside from this illness) when giving up might seem like your only option. When your health seems like a total black hole, exhausting, full of uncertainty, and blatantly shoveling dirt on top of you, this applies even more so. You might feel like you are hitting rock bottom and do you know what? That is a good thing. Do you know why? Because when you hit a bottom, you have nowhere to go but up.

My own rock bottom was not exactly a standard experience. I don't think it was obvious to many people on the outside, either. It wasn't so much that everything around me felt like it was falling apart (even though in hindsight, it totally was) or that my health was at an all-time low (again, it totally was). It was a conversation that I had with my best friend. Out of all of my friends in this experience, she was one of the few who was able to intentionally stand by me and support me in the turmoil that I was experiencing. But in this conversation, she looked at me and simply said that she was worried about me. She was worried that I wouldn't survive this because of how I was handling it all.

She was right. To hear those words come from someone else out loud shook me to my core. In a way, I had taken a path of complacency with my illness. Not intentionally, but more so out of pure exhaustion. I had gotten into a sort of routine and lacked any intention in how I was living my life between my episodes. I was just trucking along, waiting for the next attack instead of plotting how I was going to navigate my way to better health. I had completely lost my way. I knew that I had to get back to that place of strength and determination that I was sure would allow for me to heal. **I knew that I could never give up.**

An Exercise in "Why"

It was here in this profound moment that I began to think about "why" I had to do it (get better, that is). Essentially, I asked myself why exactly I felt that I needed to get better. What was I doing it all for?

Most people live their lives by focusing on *what* they have to do. The "what" makes us feel so grown up, but also so sterile. Yet when you start asking yourself "why," you almost start to feel like a child (in a good way!) Kids ask why about every. Little. Thing. I think that we all have something amazing to learn from their incessant sense of wonder. I also think that when you push to dig deeper in asking yourself about your biggest driving force in this process, you are able to discover a sense of motivation and momentum that you would otherwise not have unearthed.

Here's how to unlock your "why."

1. Write down the things that you really love to do.

2. Once you have this list, for each thing you need to ask yourself: **why you love it and why it's important to have it in your life.**

3. Make another list of the things that you hope to do someday.

4. With this list, again ask yourself **why you want to do it and why it's important that you do it someday.**

5. If you feel stuck, move on to your next thing. Chances are, if you can't come to some clarity about an item on your list with a decent amount of ease, it doesn't serve you in the way that you thought.

This process will help you to refine your lists so that they include only the things that genuinely and authentically matter to you (not just the things that sound great on the surface but have no real roots inside of your soul).

I think that if you are able to better understand your WHY, you'll have an easier time in discovering the HOW of it all. If you are not feeling motivated to take positive action in your health crisis, it might be because your "why" is not strong enough to pull you through the darkness and make you push yourself to do things when you don't feel as though you are strong enough. Your "why" can give you a tremendous amount of strength. It can give you hope and carry you through the moments that you feel like you are totally lost in a maze of uncertainty.

This is ultimately about saving your own life. It is about committing to figuring out what is wrong with you and how you can come out of the darkness to exist as you were meant to in this world. It is going to take time, hard work, dedication, and most importantly the drive and determination to get yourself and your body to a place of peace. You are capable of holding on to that light and letting it take you where you are supposed to go.

And here's the coolest part: You picked out this book because you already have this mantra inside of you. All I wanted to do in this chapter is reinforce it and strengthen its power so that it can stay at the forefront of your journey.

3. Own It

When you are placed in a situation that puts you in the minority, I think a very natural response is to want to hide. I often compare myself to a turtle in this way; any time I am threatened, emotionally or physically, my natural instinct is to retreat within myself and (attempt) to wait the turmoil out. I did this for about five out of the six years that I struggled with my health, and spoiler alert: it didn't work.

Now, I'm not talking an ownership of your illness that comes from a submissive place. There is a clear difference between ownership that consumes and ownership that gives power. **I'm talking about the kind of ownership that empowers you.** The kind of ownership in which you look your situation straight in the face and stare into its soul so that you can eventually conquer it. This is the kind of ownership that propels you forward and doesn't even give you time to think about looking back.

I lived through a majority of my experience with fortitude, but there was also a heavy dose of denial. Illness is, in many ways, a curse. But it's not without its backhanded gifts. When you have an experience like this, you are forced to find resilience and strength that you never knew you had. My denial got in the way of this for quite some time. This is where that strong sense of ownership comes into play.

The first step in this process is acknowledging that this is the hand that you have been dealt. It might not be ideal or pretty or even fair, *but it is yours*. At the same time that you acknowledge your new path, you might also need to grieve. You might need to mourn the "normal existence" that you thought you would have. This "normal" person of health no longer exists, and while that might anger or frustrate you (totally ok by the way!), I have big news for you: normal is not the vision that I have for your life.

Your (Illness) Elevator Pitch

A big issue that I had while in the thick of my fight was how I would explain my illness to others. I often found myself stuttering and embarrassed when people would genuinely ask me about what I was going through. More often than not, I stumbled through a meek response, diffused my experience and quickly changed the subject so as to avoid any further awkwardness, and that was that. I often felt defeated after this conversation and I also eventually felt like I wasn't giving people a proper chance to understand my situation and provide me with any type of support or understanding in this process.

(I'll go into more on the concept of tribe-building in later pages, but as a preface, I think that if I had mastered my own elevator pitch sooner I might have been able to receive more emotional help from others and probably not have felt as isolated throughout the process.)

In business, an elevator pitch is a quick, well-crafted (and often memorized) speech designed to sell a product, or yourself, in a very short time frame (i.e. an elevator ride). In this context, its purpose is to move another person in a powerful way so that they want to hear more even after the "elevator ride" is over.

In the case of your illness, the elevator pitch is about you. It's not so much about furthering the conversation (but of course, if it does move in that direction, go with it!), but more about helping you remain empowered in your experience. **When you can organize what you are experiencing and are able to communicate it in a way that is clear and concise, you walk away from the conversation feeling less like a victim and more like a warrior.**

The Illness Elevator Pitch also eases the anxiety of having to interact with someone new and prevents you from getting caught off guard, especially in a social setting. I can think of about a hundred situations that I found myself in where somehow my illness came up, someone was genuinely interested, I totally fumbled in my response, things got a little weird, and I left the conversation with a heavy thought: '*What if I had explained myself better?*'

Even when people are just asking to be polite and aren't really interested in providing any type of support beyond that, your elevator pitch can be a great way for you to combat their obvious disinterest in a way that becomes constructive. I had many experiences where I was trying (and probably failing) to explain my illness and the other person became obviously disinterested (or even disgusted) mid-conversation. That was tough to handle and I would take their response very, very personally. But then I realized that when you stop relying on the response of others and instead create a positive conversation within that of your elevator pitch, you are not only using it as an opportunity to educate others, but you are also creating an environment for yourself that refuses to accept even a drop of a victim mentality.

HOW TO MASTER YOUR (ILLNESS) ELEVATOR PITCH

In this type of pitch, you must do four things:

1. Clearly (but briefly) describe what is going on with your health.

2. Mention one recent stride you have made in figuring out what is going on with you.

3. Leave minimal room (if any) for a response that can, in any way, suggest that your life is depressing.

4. End with a sense of hope (and maybe a little humor thrown in there) just to relieve any potential heaviness.

EXAMPLE:

About ____ months/years ago, I started to experience these totally confusing symptoms. (You can mention 2-3 of your most prominent symptoms here if you are comfortable with that). I've seen an army of doctors and everyone is having a really tough time figuring out what is wrong with me. It's frustrating and so debilitating and it's awful to have become one of those rare medical anomalies but I have resolved to fight through this as hard as I can to find out what is going on with my health.

As of right now, my doctors are looking into the possibility that it's _____. I'm not sure where this will go, but I'm hopeful about it. I'm also doing XYZ (therapy, diet, treatment, etc.) to see if that provides any relief. It's totally exhausting but I know that at some point, we will find some clear answers. Any good vibes you have to send my way would be awesome!

Additionally, to give you an example of how your pitch can change with your situation, here's my own that I use now, almost five years into the aftermath:

When I was 17, I started experiencing these violent attacks where I would feel intense abdominal pain and basically, I would throw up for hours on end with no relief whatsoever. I spent upwards of six years going from doctor to doctor and diagnosis to diagnosis with no real break in the case. I ended up finding out that I had sphincter of Oddi dysfunction, which basically means that my body was unable to pass digestive fluids properly and this was a root cause of my attacks. By this point, my health had become such a mess and a medication that I had been taking for a while was actually perpetuating my symptoms and making my condition worse. How crazy is that? Once we started to figure this all out I also decided to take control of my health and I totally revamped my diet and lifestyle. Over time, I was able to completely take back my health and I can now say that I am happier and healthier than ever.

I often reflect on the path that I was forced to take as a result of my illness and I can honestly say that I am so grateful for it. It has given me such a powerful perspective on life that I know that I wouldn't have been able to experience otherwise. It has allowed for me to appreciate life in a way that many people can't and I'm just so thankful that I have gotten to this place of vibrant health today.

As you can see, your elevator pitch will probably always be something that you use. It will also evolve with your illness and at some point, you will use it like I do: to help others understand how you have become that strong, inspired person who has set out to do great things in life.

I heard a quote once that really stuck with me: "In life, you are either a passenger or a pilot; it's your choice." I think that if you can learn to own your situation, you are choosing strength. You are choosing to stand up instead of roll over, and you are choosing positivity in what is obviously a pretty negative situation.

You might not be able to control everything that is happening to you physically right now. But you can control how you perceive it, and further, how you react to it. Your perception of it will always be stronger than anything that it can do to or for you. Remember that. This illness, this experience (as dark and frustrating as it might be), is meant to give you strength. It is meant to change you in a way that you might not yet understand.

For years, I meekly acknowledged my illness and felt so emotionally drained because of it. I wish I had resolved to take ownership of it sooner. Bottom line: don't deny what is happening to you right now. Own it. Stare right back at it. Look it in the eye and take it all in. Let it serve you in a way that is constructive. Let it free you and inspire your path to better health.

Phase 2: AWARENESS

In this phase, you start to recognize things about yourself and others that ultimately come together to help you develop a sense of direction and stability amidst the chaos.

When you set out to become more self-aware, you begin to see aspects of your personality and behavior that you didn't notice before. **Self-awareness can help you stabilize yourself in an otherwise chaotic time and allow for you to integrate various healing practices on the path to answers and better health.**

4. No Such Thing as Normal

Before I got sick, I thought of myself in a very "normal" context. I hadn't really experienced anything that I felt dramatically set me apart from the masses of other young people and as a result, I cruised along, not thinking much about existing beyond my comfortable life. And then, when I got sick, I started to envy anyone who lived a life that didn't involve violent vomiting episodes and multiple trips to the ER every few months. It became almost hurtful to think about the hand that I'd been dealt and how it compared to others'.

Normality is, in large part, a social construct. Average is a term that society uses to group common things together in order to better explain humans and their nature. Normal, common, and average. It seems comfortable and suggests monotony. To me now, it sounds so dull! Why would anyone want to strive for things that suggest insignificance?

You might wish for your "normal" life before this but I'm going to tell you something that might sting a bit—that life of normal is not real. **No one is normal because normal doesn't exist.** It's a made up fallacy that we use as a reference point when things are happening to us that we don't like or don't understand. It's an illusion that we hold on to about what our lives *should* look like. These ideals are influenced by society, the media, friends, family and a million other things. I see the search for normal as a denial of, and resistance to, whatever is happening right here and now which results in discomfort and even pain.

People worry and feel jealousy when they try to align with normal. When you try to model your existence after something that isn't real, it can obviously prove to be a frustrating endeavor. Feelings of envy and jealousy also take valuable energy away from your main goals: to find out what is wrong with you and to get better. Your energy and this mission are two very precious commodities right now and anything that gets in the way of them should be ousted from your life as quickly as possible.

I'm not saying that it's easy to throw away the frustration and the wishful thinking. Human nature makes it tricky to ignore core feelings of desire and envy. But I think that by recognizing that normal is a total fallacy, we are better able to let go of what could have been to accept where we are now. From there, we continue to use this powerful realization to help drive through the pain and suffering to get to a place of healing.

Growing up, my mom said this phrase a lot: **We are all messed up; it's which of us get along that matters.** And it's so true. We are all a mess. We are all sloppy and trying to find our way (some more than others of course), but the point is that we are all human. We are all flawed and learning as we go. No one becomes an expert on life because by the time that you have lived a full one, you move on from this world. Instead, we all bob and weave through the ups and downs and make the best decisions that we can as we try to create the best life for our families and ourselves.

You might wish for a calm life with no surprises, but in order to live a rich, full life, you need to be willing to embrace (yes, embrace!) whatever turmoil comes your way and the bigger meaning behind it. Without any deviation from "normal," life wouldn't be the multi-textured, colorful tapestry that it really is. **The silver lining is always in this concept: the things that happen to us, even the bad things, the things that crush our normal and shake us to the core, those things are ultimately what make us better people.** They are what make us appreciate life instead of simply wandering through it. They are the things that allow for us to go deeper and become stronger, and ultimately have a positive impact on the world.

I'll take that over normal any day.

This brings me to another pivotal realization that my illness gave me about "normal" as it pertains to a medical experience. Just like society, doctors are often trained to make their assessments based on their own understanding of normal and average. This, understandably, is thought to be the best way to understand various patterns of health and illness. And while many patients do indeed fall nicely into those averages, this concept fails to address that every single human body has the very real potential to deviate outside of these "normal" boundaries. When this happens, doctors are often stumped and unprepared to handle this extraordinariness in a way that promotes a proper diagnosis and effective healing process.

When your doctor tells you that your tests look normal, my advice would be to take this with a grain of salt. I understand that "normal" is meant to assist in the process of understanding your potential condition, but what if you are that one-in-a-million person whose tests show levels of normal despite there being a very real imbalance underneath a false guise of normal numbers? What if you are that one person in your doctor's entire career who defies the numbers and manifests a particular illness in a new way?

The reality is, this could be any of us. Sickness knows no boundaries and oftentimes loves to rear its nasty little head in an atypical way. If you too quickly accept "normal" test results, especially when there are other symptoms that are pointing you in the direction of a particular diagnosis, you might miss a huge break in your case. Essentially what I'm saying is this: if you are feeling pulled toward a particular diagnosis and then you receive test results that by medical standards say otherwise, don't immediately give up on that diagnosis. Dig deeper, push farther, and listen to your gut before you let yourself be clustered into "normal".

5. Self-Awareness as a Spiritual Practice

How well your body functions depend, in part, on your emotional health. Unfortunately, many people spend years or even their entire lifetimes running from realities that seem too painful to face. Research has shown that a relentless cover-up of negative emotions exacts a distinct *physiological* toll. All the energy you expend to keep "safe" from difficult experiences leaves your body with little resilience to cope with the demands of daily life—your immune system may misfire, hormones may become imbalanced, your muscles may become chronically messed up, and your entire system may behave erratically. Even those people of "normal" health, the ones that you (used to!) compare yourself to? Their bodies are also at the mercy of their emotional existence.

On the day that I had my first attack, I experienced some very intense emotional turmoil. In short, I had my heart broken. I had never experienced these kinds of emotions before this day and anyone that has can testify to the fact that they wreak absolute havoc on you. At the time, I was 17 years old and bursting with negative anxiety. On the inside, my adolescent mind was in total shambles about it but I was trying bottle it all up so that on the exterior, no one could tell that I was hurting.

I have since had quite a bit of time to reflect on my emotional tendencies up until the moment I became sick. A big realization that I had about myself was that, for most of my childhood, I internalized nearly all of my "negative" experiences. Growing up, I went through quite a bit— divorced parents, a blended family, step-siblings who had some major issues, a move to a couple new cities, and the very tumultuous relationship and ultimate divorce of my mom and stepfather that prompted another move in the beginning of high school that totally rocked my world, both socially and emotionally.

In hindsight, all of these experiences shaped me in a way that I could not be more grateful for. They were small players in the big-picture of my life. But at the time, in the thick of it? I was big-time faking my way through it and ignoring some core emotions. Now, don't get me wrong, I reflect on my childhood and can honestly say that I was happy and that much of it was a positive experience. But I rarely, if ever, felt my feelings through the negative experiences. Instead, I denied them and I am certain that that stifled emotional state played a crucial role in my getting sick.

As I internalized these basic human emotions—grief, longing, sadness, frustration, etc.—I also became very unaware of a big part of who I was. I was detached from my own body and my own mind, trying to fake my way through it all in the hope that those unpleasant emotions would eventually disappear. Instead, they built up for years and erupted back onto me in an awful way.

Now that I am on the other side of this, I have come to a very powerful conclusion about illness: in the majority of cases, the disease or pain is the symptom—not the cause. The cause is living a life that is somehow out of balance. The illness is the body's cry for help. In my case, I was tremendously out of balance in how I processed my emotions. (Let it be said that I was also pretty of balance physically when it came to my eating habits, but I'll go into that a bit later).

In the beginning, I was so focused on my symptoms, test results, answers, treatment, the "why me?" mentality, and trying to pretend that I wasn't even sick, that I didn't take the time to reflect inward to ask myself how I got to that point in my health in the first place. I neglected to take a good hard look at what was really going on in my life, how my story was contributing, if not actually causing, the turmoil that my body was experiencing.

This imbalance can look very different across the spectrum and, without self-awareness, can go completely unnoticed or ignored for a long time. This is what happened to me. I spent the greater part of my illness adventure unable to take the idea of tuning into myself seriously. But once I did, it was THE most powerful thing! Once I began to turn on the self-awareness switch, a huge shift happened in my world—it was freeing and invigorating and I totally wish that I had let myself experience it much, much sooner.

MY PERSONAL METHODS TO SELF-AWARENESS

Use these methods to really tune into yourself:

- **Write down your dreams and goals.** It's always nice to remind yourself about the things that you want to accomplish. When you have these things physically on paper, you are able to see them more often and really feel the desire inside of you. This practice is huge in making strides—both on your illness journey and also in the big picture of your life.

- **Keep a journal.** I have always been a writer. In many cases, I am much more fluent in expressing my emotions on paper than I am in a verbal sense. I think that both are very important, but journaling has always been an amazing way for me to express all that I am feeling in a very raw, uninhibited way. The best part about writing is the ability that you can go back and reread what you write about. You can easily reflect on everything and allow yourself to dive deeper into your words to consider what they say about you and what it all means. There might be recurring themes in your writing that you start to notice, or there might be messages that hit you hard as you reread them and make you realize things about yourself. It's a really cool thing, to be able to acknowledge the power that you hold inside of you.

- **Meditation.** Meditation can be a pretty intimidating concept. I think this has a lot to do with the fact that people think that they need to be perfect at it. You might try it out and, not even 15 seconds into it, feel like your mind is wandering and you are completely incapable of silencing your thoughts. But here's the thing: you will never be a perfect meditator and this is totally fine. No one is. Meditation is all about practice and intention and allowing for your mind to exist in a calm, healing place for a fragment of time. I suggest playing around with as many apps and YouTube guided meditations as you can get your hands on so that you can really find one that resonates with you in a way that makes you want to practice it. I meditate for 5-10 minutes a day. That's all of the time that I have to give and while it might not seem like a whole lot, it has done incredible things for my psyche and my existence as a human being. Try it, please, and thank me later.

- **Which activities are having a negative impact on your health?** This one is big. It also seems a little obvious but in my case, was probably my biggest and slowest lesson learned. Denial is a powerful force and can totally blind you—but only if you let it. I mentioned before that I was trying to deny that my illness was as heavy as it was in order to cope. So I drank alcohol and ate badly and didn't exercise and had a complete and total disregard for my physical body. I thought that willpower alone might allow for me to somehow heal. Nope. You need to really get clear about the things that you are doing on a daily basis that might be contributing negatively to your story. Are you taking your diet seriously? Are you getting enough sleep? Smoking? Drinking? Are there any relationships that you are involved in that weigh negatively on you? When you allow yourself to recognize the things in your life that are not serving you positively, write them down. Put them somewhere that you will see them regularly and acknowledge them often. This prevents the denial from creeping in. In my case, alcohol was a big trigger to my illness. So often I would think, *'Oh, I can drink this time and I'll probably be fine.'* Sometimes I lucked out and the consequences weren't huge but more often than not, I paid for it big time with a nice little trip to the ER. I wish that I had been more mindful about my triggers and intentional in acknowledging them sooner. But as I always say, better late than never.

- **What are the signs that you are pushing yourself too hard?** We all have triggers. In the case of a persistent and mysterious illness, there are always things that we do that worsen or perpetuate the condition. Pushing yourself too hard, even when you are healthy, is something that will always bring your body and mind to a place of being overwhelmed. You cannot deny this fact. Believe me, I spent years trying and do you know where it left me? In a very dark and lonely place. I had to get to this place to understand why I had gotten there, but even then it was tough to admit to myself and to others that I thought that I could do too much. Be gentle with yourself. Know your limits. Recognize when you feel like you are getting to that place of burnout and respect your body enough to know that you need to scale back or slow down. For me, these signs are pretty distinct: I want to cry for no reason, I feel unexplained moments of rage, I bite my inner cheek, and I get very quiet.

In my experience, self-awareness is not so much a destination. It's more of a process. If you can allow yourself to become more mindful on an internal level, your mind-body connection can thrive and you will be capable of so much more.

6. Doctors Don't Know Everything

One of the most profound (albeit, very frustrating) revelations that I had in my experience was that doctors don't have all of the answers. I think that because they are touted as professional "experts" in their field, doctors are often placed high up on pedestals and expected to be all knowing.

Up until my illness first manifested, I had barely ever seen a doctor. Growing up, my step-dad was a physician, so the need to go elsewhere for basic care was virtually nonexistent. Aside from a knee injury and subsequent surgery, I literally have no recollection of seeing an outside doctor between the ages of 5 and 15. My point of reference on this matter was totally skewed, so it was a huge shock when I was thrown deep into the healthcare system so abruptly.

The medical system of today is technologically proficient but also very much emotionally deficient. I have always been puzzled at the "patient-centered care" mantra that floats around various healthcare institutions because, in 95% of my experiences, I was met with much inattentiveness to my needs, not only as a patient, but on a basic human level as well.

I repeatedly found myself shivering in a hospital gown, being pricked with needles and answering a barrage of skeptical questions that related to my medical history. There were absolutely times where I was met with compassion from doctors and nurses alike and I was struck by their warmth and thorough approach. These times have been imprinted fondly into my memories and I made sure to express gratitude to these exceptionally kind souls on my way out of the hospital. More often than not, though, I was taken aback by the hostility that met me at each Emergency Room entrance.

I remember each time that I arrived at the ER, filled out the paperwork, went through triage, and waited however long it took to get back and into a bed so that I could be seen. By this time, I was in agonizing pain and vomiting almost constantly, so every time I would hear the pitter-patter of feet or curtains open I would look up in the hope that this would be my moment of relief. Over time, I could almost always gauge how the rest of my experience was going to go by the look in the doctor's eye as he or she entered the room.

There is a part of me that sees where they are coming from. To them, I was a relatively fit, seemingly high-functioning young woman who had a "condition" that only occasionally swelled into an acute problem, for which a quick medicinal fix was blatantly requested. To me, my life was slowly dissolving into total anxiety and sometimes frightening pain—and ultimately the terror that it would spiral out of control (it definitely started to, by the way). I was a total mess and instead of seeing that and wanting to help me, many of them took a very cold and cynical approach.

I felt like I didn't know how to speak to the doctors with the words that would get them, as I thought of it, "on my side." Every time I came into contact with a new doctor, especially in the ER, I tried to switch up my approach—sometimes I would offer a ton of background information but I quickly learned that anything that threatens their knowledge or overwhelms them is a huge red flag. So, I tried a more minimalist-centered approach, but of course this wasted a ton of time in my effort to find relief. There is nothing more agonizing than trying to answer a barrage of basic questions about your health while doubled over in pain and vomiting continuously.

The non-ER specialists were better, but most of them chimed in to say, "You have an idiopathic problem," which is doctor-speak for "We have no clue why this is happening to you." In the absence of answers, they all started referring me back and forth to one another.

As I got passed from specialist to specialist like a total freak show, I learned pretty quickly that doctors definitely don't know everything. They are human beings and they solve problems the same way everyone else does, which means comparing the evidence (my symptoms, in this case) to their own knowledge, experience, and maybe (if you're lucky) a little research on their part. They also react the same way everyone else does when they can't come up with an answer: they look for someone or something to blame, or they send you on your way and wash their hands of your confusing condition. They move on to the next patient while you slump back into your illness.

And then there are the drugs. In the thick of my illness, I was being prescribed upwards of ten medications from multiple doctors. You name it, I likely had it in my arsenal. My friends came to know me as a walking pharmacy. At first it was funny but then it just became sad. In our first meeting, one of the doctors that ultimately helped me find answers and put me on a path to healing, told me that the first thing that he was taught in medical school was to do two things with every patient: diagnose and prescribe. From a clinical perspective, I guess this makes sense. But on a raw human level, this fails to address the reality that we are complex beings and that illness is not a one-size-fits-all situation. It is often so much more than a quick diagnosis, some scribbles on a little piece of paper, and the popping of pills. And that is where I think the medical community is failing many of us today.

The clinical approach alone doesn't work, but it's tricky because many of the brilliant minds that end up becoming very knowledgeable experts in their respective fields get there because their brains operate in a very analytic way, one that sponges up an exceptional amount of information and tries to use it to solve a host of health problems in each patient. It's difficult to fit compassion into such a systematic equation, to have that expertise pair with a genuine sense of humanity. It's often one or the other and unfortunately, this creates a huge hole in the healthcare system. Doctors and nurses see and do so much that they often become numb to the reality that every patient carries within them a deep need to simply be loved through this process.

Toward the end of my health spiral, I began to see a prestiged pain management doctor in San Diego. Because of my frequency in needing these hardcore drugs, we thought that by establishing myself with him, I would be given more credibility each time I ended up in the ER. At first, he was optimistic (read: cocky) about being able to "help" me. But this quickly turned to frustration when about three months into our relationship, as I sat there in his office, heaving into a tiny plastic bag, he looked at me and said, "Well, Rochelle, I just don't know what to do with you anymore." He wrapped up the appointment with little more than a cold shoulder shrug and a good eye roll. He was abrasive and quite frankly, disgusting in his arrogance. It has been almost six years since this happened and it still makes me physically sick to think about his insensitive behavior that day.

Doctors shouldn't be allowed to say "I don't know" and kick you out the door without a follow-up, nor should they sigh dramatically when a patient brings in a stack of tests for them to look over. A sick person shouldn't have to beg and plead for answers, much less respect, from the people who are best equipped to help them.

Let me be clear that I am not anti-doctor or anti-medicine by any means. I have spent far too much time circulating through the medical system to discredit just how well it can function for some. I have a great amount of respect for the medical professionals who *do* practice with heart. But my experience was both eye opening and discouraging, and I have brainstormed some helpful tips in how to deal with doctors.

TIPS + TIDBITS FOR DEALING WITH DOCTORS

Using these practices will best optimize your relationship with doctors:

- Good doctors want to help. You will be able to feel this. Trust your gut on this one and if you aren't getting a strong sense of compassion, it's time to move on.

- Doctors are human beings! Take your doctor(s) off a pedestal and speak to them like rational people.

- **Answer the doctor's pressing questions first.** Many doctors are so accustomed to relying on a checklist of questions that they have to get these answers before they move on. Take a deep breath, help them out and answer these questions so that you can move forward.

- **Attach a narrative response at the end of close-ended questions.** If your doctor insists on asking close-ended questions, add a narrative response at the end that may not so easily fit into a yes/no answer. (Example: It's in the middle of my chest, right here, and it started after I really pushed myself on my run tonight.)

  o Pretend that you are being asked "how" or "why" instead of "yes/no", and add your own response. Look to make sure your doctor registers this answer—does he ask you more questions to follow up on what you said? If he or she seems to ignore you, again, time to move on.

- **Ask your own questions!** Make sure that you have given some thought to the specific questions or concerns that you have before you go in to your appointments. This way you are taking full advantage of your one-on-one time and also maximizing your communication with your doctor.

- **Focus on your concerns.** If you get the sense that your concerns are being brushed over or you are not fully understanding something, politely say so. Interject with something like, "I have tried to answer all your questions, but I am still not certain my concerns have been addressed. Can you please help me understand what's going on a bit better?"

- Respect what they say and acknowledge their expertise, but don't accept this as the end-all of your information quest.

- **ALWAYS get a second opinion.** Scratch that, in this case the more opinions you have, the better (in my case, I ended up with 10+ opinions).

- **Multiple doctors NEED to communicate with one another.** Have one doctor who acts as the coordinator of your care. This doctor should keep track of all of your medications and receive notes from the other doctors that you see, so that all of your medical information is in one place and can be reviewed easily.

- If your doctor isn't supporting your fight, it's time to find a new one that will. They are out there; trust me on this!

- **If a doctor suggests in any way that you are crazy, or even subtly suggests that this is somehow an illness that exists in your head, politely end the appointment and move on to another specialist.**

In my experience, I handed over my health to physicians and to medicine in a blind act of trust and the assumption that they could (and should) figure it all out for me. In doing this,

I removed a huge source of very credible data about my own health. **Namely, myself.**

We can't treat medicine like it is magical and all knowing. The world thinks that science knows how the body works—entirely. But this amazement is also held in check by a pretty thorough understanding of how much—or how little—we know about medicine, drugs and biology. Science isn't magic, but you know what is? Science paired with compassion, intuition, determined strength, and a sprinkle of *hope*. A holistic approach to medicine is what ultimately worked for me and I think that there are many people out there who would benefit from a similar approach.

The bottom line: If your doctor is in any way giving you bad vibes, it's time to end the relationship and seek out a professional who can genuinely offer you their best support. These doctors are out there and if you need any help at all in finding them, please reach out to me personally and I will do my best to help you do so.

7. You Are Your Own (Best!) Advocate

In this process, you will become a total detective. Now that I have found my health, I am the one that friends and family turn to with any medical conundrum. It's an incredible feeling and the place that I have drawn inspiration from while writing this book.

There was a time when a doctor's word was final—his or her education and experience were considered the foundation of unquestionable wisdom. But, as I explored in the previous chapter, a doctor's expertise cannot negate the fact that they are flawed human beings, just like the rest of us. The doctor comes to an appointment with medical expertise. The patient comes in with contextual knowledge—what these symptoms mean and feel like in the broader context of their life. Communication is crucial to progressive healthcare and if you can take an active role in this process, you will ultimately be giving yourself your best shot at a vibrant life.

When it comes to your health, you need to take charge of the conversation. It is your body and your responsibility to advocate for yourself. No one else can speak for you like you can. If you don't feel like your story is being taken seriously and your concerns are going unaddressed, there is another doctor out there who is capable of giving you the time, attention, and compassion that you deserve.

It also helps to have someone close to you take on this process with you, especially if your symptoms become debilitating. In my case, my mom was right there with me on the front lines. She helped with research, brainstorming, doctor outreach, and everything else imaginable. I highly suggest that, if you are able, you bring someone on board with your situation so that they can provide you with the unique type of support needed to power through the tough, hairy spots in this process.

HOW TO BECOME YOUR BEST ADVOCATE:

Ask questions!

In regard to your health, there is no such thing as too many questions. In today's fast-paced medical system, chances are you aren't going to have a ton of time with your doctor. Make a list of questions and concerns so that you go into your appointments with a general awareness about what you'd like to achieve from the appointment. The goal here is not to challenge your doctor, but to nurture a positive and collaborative partnership with them so that everyone is on the same page and that solutions can ultimately be found. I've said this before and I'll say it again: If you are met with any disrespect or resistance on this, it's time to look elsewhere for care.

Log your symptoms.

I can tell you from experience that it's easy to assume that you will remember a certain timeline of events or cluster of symptoms, but the reality is that the chaos of your illness can fog your mind and blur your judgment in ways that you never imagined. I will also tell you that this was by far one of my weakest areas when it came to taking back my health and in hindsight, I wish I had taken it more seriously. But the good news is that I now have this incredible insight to share with you!

Everyone told me to log my symptoms and more often than not, I rolled my eyes in annoyance. I figured that I knew my body well enough, so I didn't need to take the time to tediously record everything that I ate, every emotion that I felt, every attack I had, and so forth. WRONG. Once I eventually did this, I tuned into my body and the "big picture" of what was going on. I gained a remarkable amount of perspective and intuition about what was happening to me and this awakening ultimately enhanced my recovery process.

In the case of any illness, triggers are typically involved. I mentioned before that triggers are essentially what set off your symptoms and cause the debilitating result. So, you need to track them. In my case, one of my triggers was pretty clear from the beginning: my emotions. For a while, though, I only focused on this one trigger and blatantly ignored the possibility that there were more. After a few years, I became so frustrated that I began to accept that I needed to identify if there was more to this than I originally thought. Once I began to put my lifestyle choices and symptoms on paper, I was able to see how things were really playing out much more clearly.

Brainstorm!

Never underestimate the power of a good, old fashioned brainstorming session! This fundamental approach involves strength in numbers and can be a huge catalyst in finding a solution. It's best to really dissect your symptoms here and to also take a look at your possible triggers.

- First, I recommend making a list of every symptom that you can think of. Research them separately, together, in pairs, groups, and so forth.

- Use the power of social media and/or online forums to ask if anyone has ever experienced something similar or knows anyone that has.

- Enlist a few trusted people to help you in your research. Oftentimes, different minds will notice different elements in the research process. A different perspective can be so helpful in really seeing all of the possibilities.

Understand your insurance.

Health insurance is a complicated little beast. Many of us don't fully understand the lingo written in our policies and it's easy to tuck it away in the hope that it will explain itself to you someday. It's important to empower yourself here and try your best to gain a simple understanding of your insurance policy and how it's going to ultimately affect your out-of-pocket costs as you go through treatment.

Keep ALL of your medical records together in the same place.

Technology does you a huge favor here in that it's easier than ever to electronically collect your records and store them all in one place. If you are seeing multiple doctors, they should be able to easily request records from one another. I found that this is never a reliable process, though, and it's such a time saver if you go in to your appointments with all of your records right there for the doctor to see without the possibility of a hassle. By keeping tabs on your own documents, you won't have to worry about them getting lost in the shuffle, and you can see exactly what your doctors are seeing.

Keep medical bills organized and review them as they come in.

I wish I could tell you that your medical bills will not completely overwhelm you, but chances are, you will open and collect them and experience a staggering reality: the path to good health comes with a pretty hefty price tag. In the spirit of full disclosure, my mom handled most of my medical bills and I remained fairly oblivious. In the beginning, she paid them off but over time, as my condition spiraled, we placed them on the back burner.

Once I began to come out of the fog of my illness and put myself on a path to good health, I was almost $100,000 in debt. I was not even 25 years old and 100% of these bills were medical. After processing this for a while, I decided that it would be best for me to file bankruptcy. At the time, it was the lesser of two evils and the right choice for me. I am by no means advocating that everyone do this, and I do know of other great options such as debt consolidation, so this needs to be something that you consider for yourself and only make this kind of decision after very thoughtful consideration. If you are able to, pay off your bills as they come in so that you can hopefully avoid such a dramatic financial choice.

Maintain realistic expectations.

I went back and forth about whether or not I should write about expectations. The thing about them is that they are tremendously personal and translate so differently from person to person. They often have deep roots in who we are, our past experiences, and how we have shaped our perception of the world, so to take them on can be a totally intimidating task.

When it came to my vision of a diagnosis and path to health, I see now that my own expectations were very much unrealistic. I had a belief system that I could and should exist like everyone else. Why couldn't I do the things that so many others did and experience no impact on my health whatsoever? I also saw my diagnosis in black and white. Simply put, I thought there had to be a clear diagnosis that would lead to a definitive treatment plan and that, at the end of it all, I would be cured and move along with my life as if it never happened.

But for many, there won't be a clear answer. I spent years focusing on the one "answer" to my health problems. Now that I am very much healed, I realize that there were very significant turning points in my journey that, at the time, appeared to offer a definitive answer. In those moments, I thought I had found my holy grail. But, I look back now and see that my healing process was actually the result of a cumulative effect. There wasn't one big moment, but instead quite a few smaller milestones whose sum ended up producing the human that I am today.

What I'm trying to say here is that you should be aware of expectations and allow for them to exist flexibly as you navigate this process. Allow for yourself to recognize them and use them as motivation, but try not to be discouraged if things don't turn out exactly how you thought they would.

In my experience, things unfolded very differently than I expected. And for me, different turned out to be much better than I ever imagined.

Phase 3: ACTION

You will soon find that action is the best motivation. This phase is just about that. When you start taking action, motivation follows. You might feel lethargic to your life right now. Action will help you create the momentum that you need to carry you through this trying time and beyond.

Action will help to ignite the fire that exists inside of you and it will help you start to really live your life.

8. A Natural Mindset

In the spirit of full transparency, I am now, by most standards, a total health nut. When someone has a headache, I tell them to drink a glass of water. Skin issues? I recommend probiotics. I have lived a mostly grain free and totally dairy free life for many years and I would never ever go back. I dramatically limit sugar and processed foods. Essential oils get me all giddy. Natural remedies are my go-to for everything. I eat raw garlic when I feel a cold coming on (by the way, I totally swear by this!)

I think you get the picture.

Now, I know that there is a fairly heavy stigma against people like me. And I get it. Six years ago, I very distinctly rolled my eyes at the holistic nutritionist who told me that I needed to make some dietary changes and incorporate various supplements into my regimen in order to help my body balance itself out. I scoffed at the sheer effort of it all. *There's no way I can do that!* I thought. It seemed too daunting, too unrealistic, and frankly, too hokey to work as well as she claimed it would.

So I continued on, sick and stuck and totally frustrated. About three years later, I decided to make some dietary changes. This was more out of curiosity than anything else and because I really didn't have much else to try at that point. I started small and kept at it, making gradual tweaks as I went, and do you know what happened? *I felt better than I ever had in my entire life.* Something finally clicked and I was able to see a healthy lifestyle for what it was: my new medicine.

Now, I must digress and say that I do believe in modern medicine. I believe that we, as humans, have made some incredible strides in how we treat many life-threatening (and even non-life threatening) diseases and conditions. I believe that medicine does have a *very* important place in our existence. But I believe that it is dangerously overused, even abused, and that is why I have moved so dramatically into a "natural" mindset.

It wasn't until I made very dramatic changes to my diet and lifestyle that I truly began to feel a difference inside of my body. On the outside, every skin issue that I had (acne, ingrown hairs, sensitivity) disappeared. And this wasn't just a physical transformation. My mind came to a level of clarity that, again, I had never experienced until this point. My emotions were much more balanced and regulated themselves with grace. I felt an energy that distinctly came from within, from the heart of my soul. I was happier, I felt stronger, I was able to think clearer and feel deeper. **I became alive.**

I'm not here to tell you that revamping your diet will be the end-all to your illness. I am also not here to preach to you about how you can cure yourself with a dietary change and some essential oils. What I am saying is that your body is currently experiencing a sort of war against itself. For whatever reason (and not necessarily one that you have control over), it is massively imbalanced and screaming for help. You might not have the answers that you are looking for yet, but the best thing that you can do for yourself in the meantime is to optimize your health in a holistic way so that you can give your body its best chance.

I now live by what I like to call my own Wellness Truths. These are four distinct areas that I have made significant changes in my diet and lifestyle and because of these changes I have skyrocketed my physical and emotional vitality. I can guarantee you that if you use these as a model for some of your own changes, you will feel exponentially better. Even if it's the tiniest shift, you will feel it. How do I know this? Because when you are feeling terrible, anything helps. You might not cure yourself, but in adopting these truths, you will give your body its best shot for balance and recovery. It's about optimizing what you can control in order to get to the next step.

So let's dive in to my four Wellness Truths:

#1: Food is Medicine. Food is now my go-to medicine, preventative and otherwise. The acceptance of over-processed and under-nutritional food is, quite frankly, an appalling fact of our society. How some "food" products on the shelves are even allowed to be considered food constantly blows my mind. My bottom line: I eat real, whole foods. I always buy organic when possible and when I can't, I avoid the "Dirty Dozen" produce like the plague (you can look it up; this list it super easy to find). If I can't pronounce an ingredient or can't tell you exactly what it is, I don't buy it. I drink upwards of 80 ounces of water every single day. I eat more veggies than anything else on my plate. These are my non-negotiables.

TAKE ACTION:

- Your first step is to eliminate processed foods. No more, period. No soda, no artificial anything. Just real, whole foods. *If you do nothing else, please do this.*

- If you can, I advise doing some kind of food allergy testing. This can help you gain some insight about what your body tolerates best and what might not be agreeing with it.

- When you make these kinds of changes to your diet, especially after years of eating a certain way, you must be realistic and practical. If you do too much, you won't be able to create habits that are sustainable. My advice is, unless it's a grave situation, don't make ten changes at once. Start with one, implement if for a few weeks, and then add in another.

Aim to optimize your nutrition and vitamin levels. A balance in your body creates less of a chance for any illness to wreak havoc.

#2: Exercise is Essential. Endorphins are, in my opinion, the best drug known to man. I feel a distinct shift in my mood when I do not allow myself to dive into some type of movement every single day. Sometimes, if you aren't doing something regularly, it can be difficult to know just how much of a positive impact it has the potential to have on you. If you try it, I am totally confident that you will not be disappointed.

TAKE ACTION:

- Figure out the best, most practical way that you can move your body every single day right now and do it. Maybe it's as simple as a stretch or a walk. Maybe it's a dance party by yourself or with your kids. Maybe it's a dance class with friends. Maybe it's vacuuming while listening to your favorite jams. Maybe it's a quick jog around the block. Do you love classes at the gym? Join and go! A yogi at heart? Flex your yogi toes at home or in a studio. Get a trainer or a buddy to help keep you accountable. Do whatever it takes to move your body on a regular basis.

#3: Chemicals are an Enemy (and they are everywhere). Just as I believe that medicine has its place, I believe that man-made chemicals do as well. Do you know where they DON'T belong? In our food. In our deodorant. In our makeup. In our lotions. In everyday solutions and products like hand soap and toothpaste. And yet, if you read most conventionally produced labels, there they are, plain as day (or not, they are often discretely hidden with fancy jargon) like it's no big deal that you are rubbing formaldehyde all over your body (yes, this happens!)

Most people are totally unaware that regulation over the beauty industry is minimal at best. Currently, there is no federal law that requires companies to test personal care products for safety prior to marketing them to the public. This lack of regard for public safety is appalling. I could go on about this for days, but in the name of simplicity, I am going to tell you to do your own research on this topic and educate yourself about how chemicals make their way into your everyday life.

The bottom line is this: chemicals are not meant to exist in our bodies. The exposure that we face to an array of toxic substances has the potential to do severe damage to our bodies and our health often suffers as a result. Again, do your research and inform yourself. I am also happy to help guide you in the right direction, so please reach out if that speaks to you!

TAKE ACTION:

- Again, knowledge is power! The more you know, the more that you can allow for yourself to become empowered and make the changes necessary to avoid toxic chemicals that could be contributing to your problem.

- My top easy tips:

    o Don't buy food with ingredients that you can't pronounce.

    o Buy organic! You don't want to eat pesticides. They are gross.

    o Switch all of your personal care products: EWG.org is an awesome resource for this!

    o Get natural cleaning products. I use a solution of vinegar + water + lemon essential oil every day to clean basically everything. The vinegar smell evaporates quickly and there is no risk at all for any chemical contact.

#4: Medications should be a last resort. My history with medications is slightly comical and also very, very scary. I mentioned earlier that there was a time that I had an "arsenal" of medications. I was not kidding. Here's a peek into what it looked like:

Some of it was pretty routine, like vitamins to prevent malnutrition, anti-nausea meds to help with the queasiness, and, of course, the fun that was medicinal marijuana. Some of it was straight up hard core, like the Thorazine they also use to tranquilize horses or the Dilaudid that very distinctly resembles heroin. Sometimes it was a familiar face doing something new, like Xanax, Ativan, and Klonopin, all of which work surprisingly well for nausea and totally tamed any anxiety, but also put me into a complete catatonic state and numbed me almost to my core. And then there was the Adderall that I was prescribed by a quacky psychiatrist when I complained that I was having a difficult time focusing on my schoolwork despite the fact that I was clearly taking downers that subdued all of my senses.

When I put these words onto paper and really acknowledge the scope of what I was taking, I begin to wonder how I am even alive today. It's heavy. But at the time, I was so desperate that I would take anything that had the potential to "make me better." Desperation like that blinded me to the reality of it all: that I was a total mess and a pill was never going to fix it.

I now have a very clear opinion of medicine. It can and should be used, but only as a last resort. In my opinion, you should try everything else first.

TAKE ACTION:

- Go see a nutritionist, a naturopath, a chiropractor, and an osteopath all in addition to a traditional MD. Broaden the scope of your hope for health and really exhaust all options before you take any prescription medications.

9. Get Yourself Together

Your Relationships

I've mentioned before that for years my approach to my illness was very much about pretending that I wasn't sick. But I was, so to say that my approach was flawed is an understatement. I experienced a dissolution of so many friendships, either directly at the hands of my illness or as a byproduct of my denial.

Having the support of your entire circle is a fantasy for most patients, especially when it comes to invisible and mysterious illnesses. At the time, I took it all so personally. When you are experiencing something that starts to consume your life, it's frustrating when those around you seem oblivious to your turmoil. The envy kicks in and a cycle perpetuates:

hope → denial → envy → frustration → repeat

As I denied the heaviness of my situation, bottling it all in, the frustration built inside of me. I was essentially an emotional ticking time bomb with a super short fuse. Anything would set me off. I drank. I partied. In addition to my arsenal of prescription medications, I dabbled in recreational drugs too. I cringe now at my total inability to cope and the choices that I made as a result.

Between the ages of 17 and 23, I didn't have any social clarity about my illness. First of all, I had no idea what my illness even was, and second, I really had no idea who *I* was either. This was a terrible combination. I didn't understand that it wasn't appropriate to lead with my illness on a date or to ask just anyone to take me to the ER. I didn't know whether to pretend that it wasn't happening, go all in and tell them everything, defend myself, force them to read my medical history, or completely throw them out of my life. And everyone responded differently, making this a very unpredictable experience.

With a few exceptions, my close friendships followed a fairly distinct pattern: become super close, go all in and open up about my illness, assume that they would totally understand and embrace it, experience a weird and awkward trial when they somehow went about their own life and seemingly disregarded the heaviness of my situation, and finally, an explosion that came about after weeks of tension and my hurt feelings. End of friendship. Devastated, I would pick up and move on. I cited their inability to handle my illness as the reason for the "breakup" and it took me years to figure out that it really wasn't them. ***It was me.***

It's easy (and normal, by the way!) to get distracted by fears, ego-obsessions, drama (in your own life and in the world), ambitions, and all sorts of survival instincts and emotional reactions. But when these distractions happen, you aren't able to fully engage in what is most important: saving your own life. You need to be proactive and focus on the relationships that truly matter in this season of your life. It might be difficult to do this, given your situation, so I've come up with a few revelations to help guide you through this process.

Revelation #1: It's okay if people don't understand.

It's okay if people don't get it. This doesn't necessarily mean that they are bad relationships or bad people. We live in a totally self-absorbed society and the reality is, we are all trying to find our own way. We are all fighting a battle or on a mission, and while it's totally reasonable for you to expect support, you need to know that you might not always get it.

Revelation #2: You are who you surround yourself with.

You are the average of the people that you surround yourself with. Take inventory of the people in your life right now. In a perfect world, all of your friends and loved-ones would get it and jump on board with your fight. When people don't, it breaks your heart and drags you down. Right now, you need people who are capable of lifting you up and helping your cause, so it's important to keep close contact with those who are capable of emotionally supporting your mission and your fight to get better.

This doesn't necessarily mean that you need to dramatically cut people from your life, but you need to be conscious of how your relationships exist and can and have the potential to play into your illness. If a relationship has a negative undertone in any way, it's best to acknowledge this fact and remove yourself from it.

Revelation #3: You can put relationships on hold.

You might not have the time or the energy to sit down and evaluate exactly how you are going to approach every single relationship that is not serving your quest for a solution. I know that it can also be scary to think about cutting people out of your life when your world feels like it's getting smaller and smaller from your illness every day.

You can, by all means, place them on hold (physically, emotionally or both) so that you can address them later on, when you are emotionally and physically capable of putting energy into that process. Keep in mind, too, that people change. Someone who might not support you today could easily reach out and offer their hand in support tomorrow.

Revelation #4: You must forgive the relationships and the people who are unable to serve you in this season of your life.

Right now, you are in a very trying season of your life. It is one that requires your full commitment, attention, and strength. It's one that requires you to give all that you have to yourself and to forgive all else other than that fact. Your energy is best spent on solving and healing, not worrying about others. Eventually, you will find the strength to stand up for yourself and ask for people in your life to separate your illness from your personality.

Your Soul

When your future is threatened, it can be difficult keep your head above water. It dominates every conversation. It invades every thought. It totally stresses you out. You feel like you don't know how to handle it. It's easy to become weary and tired of carrying the burden.

You were born to contribute to this world. Every single human being has the potential for great impact. Whatever you do, don't let this hurdle drown out the work you are meant to do beyond this experience. Think about what drives you and what motivates you. What are your goals in life? What are your big dreams? What is your vision for yourself and for your life? With a little time and soul-searching, you might be able to see the exciting destination vividly, but, given the circumstances, you have a lot of doubt about how to move forward.

Fact: Getting clear about what your soul craves and your life goals can help you in your darkest times.

In addition to vibrant health, my soul has always craved connection and creation. I dreamt of meeting the love of my life and starting a family. I dreamt of the day that I would become a mom and have the privilege of raising cool little human beings. For me, that was the "thing" that I was born to do. That was the moment that I was living for.

That moment would ultimately prove that in the face of this illness, I had won. Never once did I lose sight of this dream. I always acknowledged this desire, no matter how unrealistic it seemed to anyone on the outside. I knew that someday, somehow, I would get there.

An Exercise in Positive Words (aka Affirmations)

I've already mentioned how powerful the mind is, but it's always worth exploring more.

Affirmations are positive statements or thoughts that you consciously focus on in order to produce a desired result. In other words, it is a very focused way of positive thinking. Affirmations can be whatever you desire but the trick here is that you must firmly believe that what you are telling yourself is true.

Traditionally, affirmations tend to involve telling yourself something that might not be true in this moment, but you aim to get there at some point. I understand this approach, but it never fully resonated with me. I think that in this specific type of situation, these perfection-based affirmations can be overwhelmingly discouraging and create more negativity and frustration than anything else.

Here's what I'm talking about: typically, in the case of a person's troubled health, a suggested affirmation might go something like, 'I am healthy' or 'I am healed.' The theory here is that if you tell yourself that you are healthy frequently enough, it will become so. The mind is probably the most powerful weapon that you have here, but let's be real: telling yourself that you are healed while you are curled into a tiny ball in pain is probably going to piss you off more than anything else.

When you are sick, struggling, and feeling that physical and emotional burden every day, it's nearly impossible for affirmations like these to resonate with how your life exists right now. You can tell yourself that you are healthy until you're blue in the face, but the reality is that you are having a tough time and you need to *own this* in your affirmations in order for them to be effective.

I prefer a more realistic approach to this process, one that is fueled by hope. *I prefer positive words that are real,* not necessarily ideal.

Affirmations can be tricky. I have spent years working on my own and let me tell you, I don't think that they ever become "perfect". But, here are some really basic and really great places to start:

I can _____.

I will _____.

I believe _____.

My body can _____.

_____ is possible.

I commit to _____.

I am strong, I am alive, I am _____.

I CAN DO THIS.

Some great words to fill in the blanks here: heal, healing, find health, strong, power, balance . . . I think you get the picture.

Some helpful guidelines:

- Use words that lift you up. For me, words like vibrant, thrive, and strength, are ones that really get me going and speak to the fire in my soul.

- Avoid negative words. For example, if you were to say, "I am not sick" you would be using two negative words. The word "not" has a negative context, just as sick does. You are not on a mission to deny what is happening to you, but instead, combat it with those uplifting and empowering words.

- Gratitude is a powerful force on its own. Be grateful for every little thing in your life and give thanks for your affirmations. "Thank you for my hope," and "Thank you for my strength," are great places to start.

- You need to believe in what you are saying! Feel the hope, feel the energy, feel the positivity as you say them.

Instead of seeing this challenge as a problem, there is a far more effective way to address the illness that threatens your big picture dreams and appears to be holding you back: **turn it into an ally.** If you can reframe the way that you see your illness, you can channel that strength into something totally powerful, something that will end up really resonating with your soul.

I know this concept might be strange to put into practice and quite frankly, it blatantly defies most common, rational sense. What I'm talking about here though is your perspective. It's about allowing yourself to embrace what you are experiencing and know that on the other side of this you will be stronger, more aware, more grateful, more empowered, and more alive because of it (both inside and out). This right here, this is the place that it becomes your friend.

Toward the end of my experience, I tried to think about how I was going to collaborate (yes, collaborate!) with my situation in order to use the negative experiences and circumstances to make myself better (again, both inside and out). I sought out to really train my mind to not feel that negative jolt of energy whenever I would think about or talk about what I was going through. I'll be honest and tell you that this was not an overnight process. It took months of consciously reframing my perspective before I was able to get myself to a place where the negativity was no longer my default.

My biggest tip for this process is to use positive words as much as you can, just as you would use your affirmations. Personally, I found gratitude to be my most powerful method of shining a positive light on my situation. I made a very conscious effort to immediately practice gratitude for my illness whenever I thought or spoke about it.

I'm grateful that it gave me such a powerful perspective on life. I'm grateful that it taught me how to become my own advocate. I'm grateful that it showed me the true value of good health. I'm grateful for the fact that I was ultimately able to make moves toward a place of healing. I'm grateful that it made me totally and completely appreciate every single breath that I take.

Gratitude allowed me to make this illness my ally. It is now the biggest driving force in how I live day in and day out. I would be lying if I told you that those negative emotions are no longer there. Every now and then, they creep back in and

I shudder at the thought of what I went through. But I think that this is more of a good thing. It's a humbling reminder of where I came from and why I live so intentionally now.

10. Feel Your Feelings

"Human beings are emotional creatures first, rational creatures second."

—David Julio Wang

Men and women are very different creatures but when we think about emotional capacity, we both tend to bottle our feelings in some way. For men, this comes from a stoic, masculine place of denial. For women, it comes from a place of protection—protecting others around them from the reality of their feelings. For everyone, this bottling also generally comes from a place of wanting to avoid some type of judgment.

It can be so much easier to bottle up your emotions than it is to face them. Often, the pain that they hold seems like it's too much, too deep or too damn scary. This is called **emotional suppression**—an emotional regulation strategy. Emotional suppression is the deliberate or conscious avoidance or pushing away of thoughts or feelings to cope with trauma. It is something that many of us do to make uncomfortable thoughts and feelings more manageable.

Emotions are a part of life and can oftentimes be painful, but suppressing them doesn't work. In fact, it can typically make things worse. Have you ever tried your hardest to avoid thinking about something, only to become quickly annoyed with the fact that you actually seem to think about it more? This is what I'm talking about here.

Your emotions eventually affect your beliefs, standards, and habits. They influence the goals you set for yourself and whether or not you achieve them. When you internalize your emotions, they don't go away. Instead, your body absorbs them. In my case, I had been internalizing my emotions for *years*. (I was internalizing both positive and negative experiences, by the way!) But where did this come from? After quite a bit of reflection, I have linked it back to my need to put on a happy face at all times, no matter what. I do this to protect myself and while my intentions are good, the end result is not.

That stoic, mannequin approach is not sustainable long-term. It creates a mind-body disconnect that slowly eats away at your insides and eventually has the potential implode your physical health. **You need to give yourself permission feel your feelings.** All of them. The happy, the sad, the angry, the frustrated, the confused, the empowered, the excited, and everything in between.

This kind of emotional self-care is crucial to you finding the balance within your body that you are looking for. In this journey, you will likely experience a very overwhelming scope of emotions. Some of them will be directly related to your illness and many others will likely be the result of whatever else is going on in your life. Feel them all. Open your arms and your heart and allow yourself to see them, touch them, taste them, hold them, smell them, and eventually, to release them instead of sucking them back into your physical body.

Once I gave myself permission to exist as the emotional being that I am wired to be, that we are all wired to be, I began to see how my emotions were engaging with my illness. They were distinct triggers in my attacks and a pretty clear pattern emerged, but I was clueless on how to implement any constructive regulatory practices into my routine.

I had finally acknowledged that I was internalizing my emotions, but where to go from here? Over time, I experimented with various forms of release. These are the methods that I found to be the most helpful:

- *Accept your emotions on a level that is free of judgment.* Don't dwell on them or beat yourself up. They are what they are, nothing more and nothing less. You're not what is happening to you. Be gentle with yourself.

- *Talk to yourself.* I am that person who LOVES to talk to myself in the car. I find it tremendously therapeutic to verbally release my emotions into the world, all in the safety of a small, enclosed space where no one else can hear me or judge my feelings. I encourage everyone to try it!

- *Journal.* Writing is another therapeutic medium that can provide a wonderful release of emotional build up. I love that when I write I'm able to organize my thoughts and emotions and fully express them. At first it feels like a total emotional mind dump, but eventually I use my writing to craft words and a voice that eventually works toward empowerment.

- _Open up to one (trusted) person_. This can be tough, but you do eventually have to dive in and open up to another human being. This connection is so important to the basic fundamental human needs that we all have. This person can be someone that you already know or it can be a total stranger (likely in the form of a therapist). It really doesn't matter how you decide to seek this connection—what's important is that you cultivate it in order to best address and process your feelings and emotions.

- _Exercise!_ One word: endorphins. No explanation needed here. Move your body in whatever way that you can!

Like it or not, our emotions play a role in every single thing that we think and do. You are allowed to be emotional (obviously as you navigate this experience, but also outside of it as well!) **Feelings often have far more influence over us than all the rational, logical thought in the world.** So instead of falling victim to them, I like to choose to use them in a way that is constructive (once I've acknowledged and felt them, of course). Our emotions have the power to spark a mission, create momentum, and allow you to let that fire inside of you forge gold for your life.

11. Do Your Homework

Knowledge is power.

I've already explored the fact that, throughout this process, you will (if you haven't already) master the role of a detective. The research process plays a HUGE part in this so I wanted to address my own experience.

Just about anyone with internet access and a body that occasionally goes haywire has had the experience of Googling their symptoms and watching, horrified, as the results stream in. It's a well known fact that Dr. Google can very easily make you think that awful things are happening inside of your body that, realistically, are probably not. Headache = brain tumor! Sharp pain in your side = punctured lung! Sore post-workout legs = deep vein thrombosis! Millions of medical sites, blogs, and Wiki pages can, intentionally or not, spew out confusing, overwhelming, or panic-inducing information—or, in too many cases to count, *mis*information.

Because of this, many people will tell you not to Google every single little thing. And if you were someone experiencing everyday ailments that weren't all consuming, I might tell you to ease off of the computer so as not to induce an anxiety attack. But you are experiencing something perplexing and complicated, so in my opinion, the more that you can find out, the better.

I say, Google the hell out of your symptoms.

The internet is quite possibly one of your greatest health tools. It has the ability to connect you with ideas and experiences and people from all around the world. When you are fighting an illness and no one has been able to give you answers, you need as many outside, unique connections as you can get. Doing some homework can absolutely jump-start your healing process.

The key here is to not go into an internet search putting blind trust in Dr. Google. You're not necessarily looking for the answer (although you very well might find it). You're looking to arm yourself with as much knowledge as possible in this matter. In my opinion, the more that you know about your own body and your symptoms, the better that you can educate yourself and your doctor on any of the possible solutions that speak to you with potential.

All it takes is that one idea to spark a solution. The smallest, most insignificant of symptoms can actually give you a break in the case. And let's face it, you're totally going to Google everything anyway, so I might as well give you a few key tips that helped me navigate the internet without experiencing being totally overwhelmed.

Here's how to not go crazy while consulting Dr. Google:

Keep in mind that not everything on the Internet is accurate. This one might seem like a no-brainer, but it's important to start here. Particularly when you are acting in slight (or total) desperation, it can be easy to see any potential informational help with rose-colored glasses. I get it. I was there. I think that it helps to go into this more with the intent of finding the catalyst to the solution of the illness rather that the "name" of the illness itself. Set your expectations low and aim to empower yourself with knowledge, more so than finding clear and distinct answers.

Patient persistence is your best friend. I can think of at least three potential diagnoses that, at the time, I was SURE would lead to my "cure". I wanted them to be "my cure" so badly that I ignored any other potential diagnoses for a good chunk of time after that. I'm not saying that this time was wasted, but I wish that I had been able to allow myself to take in the information, process it, and reflect about whether or not it really applied to me. But hindsight is 20/20, so all that I can say is, no matter what, patience + persistence = your greatest hope for answers and health.

***Always* consider the source.** Is it reliable? Was the content medically reviewed? Is the information reported elsewhere? If you can't verify the information through another source, definitely question it and dig a little deeper before forming an opinion.

Consult reputable medical sites. Sites like www.MayoClinic.com and www.Health.gov can help you gain professional insight into how your symptoms might fit together.

Don't self-diagnose. This one can be so tricky! Your consultation with the internet shouldn't be so much about a diagnosis as it needs to be about becoming as educated as possible. Your ultimate goal should be to use the Internet constructively to research your symptoms and the possible conditions they can lead to in order to come up with questions to ask your doctor(s).

Look beyond your symptoms! Be sure to keep track of medications and supplements that you are taking, research them all and know what you're dealing with here. Drug side effects and conflicts are oftentimes worse than the original condition and can totally complicate your efforts. In my case, I ended up with a situation that was compounded by the fact that I was taking too many drugs that shouldn't have been taken together, one of which was definitively perpetuating my illness. The combination of prescriptions made a mess of my body and my health and it became difficult to know whether or not my symptoms were real or simply a byproduct of medicinal side effects.

Research specific doctors who might be able to help. There may be experts who are researching sets of symptoms that don't even have a name yet. If you dig deep enough, you'll likely be able to find doctors or researchers who seem to be working on ideas related to your mystery illness. Find an email address for those people and contact them directly.

The very illness that I ended up having was the direct side effect of a medication that I was taking to treat it. I was literally in a spiraling cycle. Over ten doctors overlooked it before I came into contact with one who knew about this side effect. This particular doctor specialized in pain management and drug dependence recovery. He's not the type of doctor that I initially thought I would need to see, but his specialty ended up being a catalyst in my recovery. Don't ever limit your scope of doctors.

If you have a hunch, follow it. Your illness knows no boundaries and when it comes to specialists, you should never limit yourself.

Phase 4: ADAPTATION

In this phase, you learn to recognize and restructure your life patterns and perceptions. Everything in life is fluid. Change can be hard, but it is so good for the soul.

Just as it's important to be strong in this process, it's also crucial that you remain flexible.

Adaptation means that you are figuring out how to thrive in this world.

12. Build Your Ark

Regardless of your religious affiliation, you likely have at least a bit of familiarity with the story of Noah's Ark. Essentially, this ancient allegory is one of survival and endurance and can be used as a model for your perseverance in this situation well beyond its traditional, faith-based sense.

For those of you who aren't familiar with the story, let me give you a quick rundown:

A long time ago, there was a man named Noah. According to the bible, he was the only man with integrity left in the world and because of this, God wanted to start over. He told Noah to build an ark and to prepare for a great flood that would wipe out all living things. He told Noah to gather two of every animal and make sure that he and his family joined these animals in the ark when the rain began. God also told Noah that he could include anyone that understood what he was doing and believed in his mission. No one did, and so they all perished in the flood while Noah and his family remained safe and went on to repopulate the world.

Now, I probably need to add a disclaimer here that I do not wish for your unsupporters to die in a great flood. What I do want to say, though, is that you need to build an emotional (and partly physical) ark of your own. Your illness is like the great flood. This ark will help you carry yourself through it.

HOW TO BUILD YOUR ARK

Follow these methods to help build up your best support system:

- **Get organized.** It wasn't raining when Noah started building. He was acting on faith. The idea here is that you need to get clear about where you want your future to go and actively take steps in order to get there. The more jumbled that you are in this process, the more overwhelming it will feel. Become physically organized in terms of your record keeping, new research, doctors, specialists, experiences, and so forth.

- **Ignore your critics.** I know this one can be tough, but in the context of your illness (as well as in life), criticism is a negative force that has the power to weigh heavily on you and deter you from your end goal. If you do anything with criticism, let it be that it motivates you to prove that your critics are wrong. My biggest piece of advice? Listen to your heart. Take action based on what your heart tells you, not how peer-pressure or judgment makes you feel. You are not just a part of the crowd. You are an individual on a mission. Stay on course.

- **Own who you are.** You are the most influential person in your life and this means that you are ultimately the secret to your own success and happiness.

- **Take care of yourself.** Stay physically, mentally, spiritually, and emotionally fit. Be mindful of things that trigger you and do your best to weed them out. Essentially, you are being asked to do something really big here, so this journey will require you to take the very best care of yourself in the process.

- **Handle this adversity with grace and strength.** In times when you feel unable to fight and unable to get away, do your best to stay afloat in the storm until you can get your bearings. More people fail in life as a result of internal conflicts and adversity than because of external conflicts and adversity. When you have self-awareness, you can master your inner conflicts from a position of power instead of becoming its victim.

- **Your emotions are fuel.** All of your emotions are valid and, if you let them, can play a productive role in this process. Your emotions can fuel either positive or negative actions, or they can be buried. To deny an emotion or use it in a negative space is a huge waste of your time and energy.

- **Action is the best motivation.** I've said this before, but this one is so worth mentioning again. The experts can absolutely help you find a diagnosis and a solution but all of it starts with you. Your actions give off so much more in the way of energy than your thoughts, so if you can get to a place where you are consciously and purposefully able to take action, shifts can happen and doors can open for you.

- **Your ark is your opportunity.** And opportunity often presents itself in unexpected ways. If you can build yourself a cushy lifeboat, then you are obviously positioning yourself to best handle this challenge. But do you know what you are also doing? You are preparing for what's on the other side of this.

- **Hold tight to optimism.** Your faith—in whatever it is that speaks to you—is your beacon of light. No matter how dark or overwhelming it gets, you need to know that there is always a rainbow on the other side of this storm.

13. Build Your Tribe

"No man is an island, entire of itself; every man is a piece of the continent, a part of the main."

—John Donne, Devotions upon Emergent Occasions

A tribe, also known as a pack, clan, elected family, posse, crew, network, or true friends, is basically just a group of people who share common interests and values, and most importantly, a genuine appreciation for each other. **Your tribe members are those people who accept you just as you are, and who want the very best for you.** They make you feel understood, they encourage you, and inspire you to do great things. Most significantly here, the members of your tribe help you through the difficult times. They provide you with a sense of community and support and combat any sense of isolation that you may feel in this frustrating experience.

Before this illness, you might have already felt like you existed as part of a tribe. For whatever reason, when you became ill, some or all of the members of your tribe were not able to understand or embrace what you are dealing with in this moment. Many people have a hard time wrapping their heads around this type of situation, so they either run away or pass judgment. The hurt that you feel is like nothing you've ever experienced in your life. It's heavy and messy and probably makes you feel angry and hurt.

You need to know this: Just as we humans constantly evolve, so does our tribe.

Without a solid tribe, you might feel lost, depressed, lonely, frustrated, resentful, or even scared. Human nature naturally craves intimacy and belonging. When you begin to feel deprived of these basic needs, your body responds on an emotional level that can eventually translate further into your physical well-being. Copious scientific data proves that loneliness is a greater risk to your health than smoking or lack of exercise, and finding your tribe has the potential to supplement your health better than any vitamin, diet, or exercise regimen.

At the end of the day, you need people who get you and love you and support you and who will lift you up to fight this health crisis with you. We were never intended to fight battles like this by ourselves. Your tribe will give you more energy and strength than you could ever possibly have alone.

As it relates to your illness, your tribe can play a very important role in your mindset, which ultimately factors into the healing process. The people who band around you in support are almost acting as your preventative medicine and your lifeboat all at the same time. On an emotional level, you will feel connected with your tribe. You will feel supported and empowered, and that is an essential system that must exist in order for you to come out of this in a way that is productive. For you right now, positive support is essential. The people who can't support you at this time need to be replaced (for now, at least) by people that shine light into your darkness.

Think of it this way: The people you surround yourself with have a huge impact on every aspect of your life. These people affect how you see yourself, how you feel, how you fight, and eventually, how you win this battle. They will help to shape your journey now, through this process, and far beyond it. They ultimately impact who you become and how you exist after this experience.

Going further, we have a subconscious tendency to model the behavior of those around us. You need to focus on choosing a tribe that is strong, positive, empowering, and totally believes in you, your mission, and your fight. If you set out to choose your tribe consciously and constructively, their positivity will directly reflect on how you exist, particularly in this season of your life, but also into the next.

So how does one go about building a tribe like this?

1. **Write down what this tribe looks like.** If you don't get clear about who these people are, it's going to be very difficult to find (and keep) them. I find that is really helpful to outline the types of people that you are looking for in order to stay true to yourself and this mission that you are on. It's also super helpful to have this as a point of reference any time that you feel overwhelmed or lost in this process. Ask yourself, *'what defines my tribe?' 'What are the elements that make us who we are?'* The more honest you are here, the better. A sample "tribe" looks something like this:

   I am looking for people who are able to accept my health crisis free of judgment. These people won't make me doubt myself or feel like there is something wrong with me. They will radiate positivity and empowerment, and help to lift me up when I feel lost or defeated.

This is a pretty basic start and you can get as specific as you want here. My advice is to try your best to keep your heart open to any relationship that you feel serves you positively.

2. **Seek them out!** Use <u>any</u> method that you can think of to do this. Some ideas include:

   - Online support groups

   - Local Meetup groups

   - Social media

   - Local classes that interest you (yoga, art, dance, food, etc.)

   - Community events

Some of the "lay people" in these groups (mainly the ones that focus on community in the face of illness) are way more knowledgeable than many doctors! They have so much to offer you in the form of encouragement, compassion, and genuine concern for your journey and suffering. Support groups can also be a really awesome place to connect, share, laugh, serve, and not feel alone. Keep in mind, though, that you don't necessarily need to focus on meeting people who are illness-focused. Even someone who has no idea what you are going through can shine a really positive light into your world and uplift you in many ways. It's all about meeting *positive people.*

3. **Engage.** Once you find them, you need to nurture a relationship. As much as you might hope, no one is going to go out of their way to offer love, guidance or support unless you actively participate in creating a bond. Be authentic in who you are, why you are reaching out, and what you hope to gain from the relationship.

4. **Listen to your inner voice and trust your instincts.** When was the last time you had a gut feeling about someone? Sometimes you'll meet someone new and you'll feel drawn to them right away, almost as if you were old friends. Other times you'll come across people who might appear to be the type you are looking for, but something inside of you immediately makes you want to put up your guard. Listen closely to your gut reaction to others and adjust accordingly.

5. **Help others.** It might seem like a daunting task, but if you can offer something to someone else (in the form of advice or even just a smidge of emotional support and kind words), I guarantee that you will feel better and feel like you are really a participant of your tribe.

6. **Do things with your tribe.** This doesn't have to be an overwhelming event! It can be as simple as chatting about what is going on with each of you. For members who live locally, it can be a coffee date or a walk in the park. Have regular meals together if

possible (food is a fantastic bonding mechanism!). For virtual members of your tribe, it might be as simple as a short and sweet email every now and then. This doesn't have to be a time consuming experience and can be very so simple. Do whatever speaks to you and don't worry about being perfect here. Just take action and let the rest fall into place.

In my experience, there are three key benefits from building your own tribe as you endure this health crisis:

1. Everything feels more real. When you connect with your tribe, you have the emotional and mental space to be authentic. You have nothing to prove to anyone, and that in and of itself is incredibly freeing. You'll be allowed to express your true feelings and your situation will generally feel more fluid (in this case, movement forward is always a good thing!) Just as you will feel more real, so will your illness. Oftentimes, denial is our first defense mechanism (it was mine, one hundred percent). If you surround yourself with people who don't deny that you are sick but instead help you focus on how you can get to a solution, this helps you to prioritize what you need to do and the mindset that you need to have in order to get there.

2. You feel inspired (with and without them). When you are around a supportive crew, you feel good about who you are, illness and all. You become hopeful and inspired to be the best you that you can be, which propels you to take the best care of yourself, your body, your mind, and your soul. A solid tribe engages in heart-warming conversations and fosters actions that are positive. What's even better is that you'll feel empowered even when you are not around your tribe. This "residual glow" is something that you can take with you everywhere. You'll leave them with more spring in your step, more smiles, and a strong burning internal fire. These good tribe vibes are crucial to your journey through this illness and also, of course, into the aftermath.

3. More Knowledge = More Power. The more people that you are able to genuinely make a connection with, the more experience that you can all draw from, the more ideas come to light, the more productive brainstorming sessions you are able to have, more researching happens, and so forth. Strength in numbers, people. It's one of the oldest expressions in the book and there's a reason it's so pervasive in society. A collaborative approach is one that naturally manifests strength.

The members of your tribe are ultimately your allies in this journey. When you set out to create or expand your tribe, look for people who will lift you up, help you grow, recharge you, inspire you, celebrate with you, and who are genuinely willing to be there for you when you need it. Beyond these guidelines, you need to remember that as a tribe member you do have a sense of emotional responsibility toward this tribe that you create. Make it a point to give back to the tribe and offer other tribe members your support in any way that you can.

I have one more super important tip for tribe building that I think often goes ignored: **The numbers don't matter here.** At all. Your tribe can be two people or it can be twenty. Quality over quantity plays heavily into your life now. Focus on the depth of your relationships, not the numbers. If you are lucky enough to have one understanding and inspiring friend in your circle, hold tight to them, respect what they are graciously able to offer you, and make sure that you are mindful and grateful in every interaction that you have with them.

Ultimately, your tribe can save your life and make it feel like it is really, truly possible to conquer this battle.

14. The Diagnosis

You might be desperate for a diagnosis, and it's easy to take the first one that comes along in the hope that this will be your big break. I mentioned that I was totally here and I know what it's like to feel that desperation and spring on the first answer that comes your way. Medical purgatory is awful, especially with a diagnosis you may or may not believe and treatments that aren't working (and even if they are, they aren't getting to the root cause). And then there's you, the patient, who has become so debilitated (physically and emotionally) that it becomes truly difficult to see or believe that there is any way out.

In some cases, the problem isn't that you're unable to get a diagnosis. The problem is that you've received an inaccurate one. If your treatment isn't making you feel better, don't immediately look for other therapies. Your first move should be to confirm that your doctor got the diagnosis right in the first place.

This is where the idea of a Differential Diagnosis comes into play.

Clinically speaking, a differential diagnosis is the distinguishing of a particular disease or condition from others that present similar symptoms. When it comes to an illness that is tough to crack, this concept can be pretty huge.

Essentially, every doctor uses clues (drawn from your descriptions of symptoms, your medical tests, and their own knowledge of medicine) to make a list of all the possible diagnoses that could explain what is medically wrong with you. Then, one by one, using those same clues, he or she will begin to narrow down the list by finding clues that don't fit.

Typically, a differential diagnosis refers to an actual diagnosis. But what if you are unable to receive that? Ask your doctor:

- "What can it be?"

- "What are the possibilities?"

- "What else can it be?"

These questions can make a major difference in your care because it's important for you to know what those other potential diagnosis options were/are, and why they were eliminated. You can use them to gain important insight into what's wrong with you as you endure this process.

Write down the names of any diagnoses your doctor suggested or rejected. Later, if the treatment you choose doesn't seem to be working, you may wonder if you have been misdiagnosed. Knowing what your diagnosis' possibilities and alternatives were can help you and your doctor hone in on a more accurate answer later, if necessary. You can also try to find a diagnosis using a different perspective: a backwards approach, if you will. Start with your least common symptoms and move from there.

Your opinions should also come from a variety of resources. In particular, avoid doctors who practice together or who may be friends outside the office or hospital. Friends and colleagues may be less likely to disagree or contradict each other. The professionals who work in academic medical centers (university-related hospitals) can be really great sources for solving your diagnosis dilemma because their personal and professional goals are sometimes better aligned with your needs.

15. It Takes a Village

Sometimes it takes more than just the people around you to come to a diagnosis. Building your tribe is a great place to start, but if you find yourself still needing help/input/answers, you need to think big. We are lucky to live in a world where we can instantly and regularly connect with people who are thousands of miles away from us. The theory here is simple: the more people that you connect with, the higher your chances of finding someone who has experience with a similar situation. The more people that you reach, the better your chance of finding the spark that can ignite your path toward healing.

I personally used this tactic and found a very knowledgeable doctor in Milwaukee, Wisconsin who ended up mentioning that I could have a rare form of sphincter of Oddi dysfunction (see the Preface for more specifics on this if you're interested). This general potential diagnosis had been brought up before, but I had already undergone a procedure to go in there and check it out, and it looked totally fine. Typically, when someone has this condition, the sphincter of Oddi becomes blocked or closes off and stays that way. Her thought was *maybe* in my case, it was spasming in an attack, relaxing and then reopening. This could explain why, since I had the investigative procedure in a time when I was not directly in an attack, the results came back "normal". She mentioned that she had seen this happen only once before in her career but that it was very much in the realm of possibility.

So, I came back to San Diego and found a specialist locally who had experience with sphincter of Oddi dysfunction. (If you read My Story in the beginning of this book, I also mentioned this there as well.) Though he had never seen it himself, he agreed that this new theory was possible and we decided to go ahead and put a tiny little stint (kind of like a door stop) in the opening of my sphincter of Oddi for a period of time so we could see if I noticed a reduction in my attacks. And I did. It felt like a full-blown miracle. So about six months later he went in and performed a sphincterotomy (basically, he cut my sphincter of Oddi open so that, even if and when it does spasm, my fluids are not affected and there is no buildup and thus, no attacks). From there, my journey was far from over but a root cause of my illness had been taken care of. This was a huge breakthrough!

All because I went in search of a doctor outside of my little bubble. It's amazing what can happen when you reach beyond what's comfortable.

Some additional tips:

- Look for doctors around the country and even the world. Don't limit yourself *at all*.

- Some of the best, most innovative specialists can be found at large hospitals or, better yet, at teaching hospitals affiliated with medical schools.

- It's especially important to seek this top level of expertise once you've seen and/or stumped other doctors.

- Doctors at a university center usually have the most up-to-date information on rare diseases, and they have an array of specialists that can address them.

- *CrowdMed*—For people who are experiencing something mysterious, this site allows patients to submit their cases to be solved by a group of "medical detectives" from around the world. I never used this but some amazing success stories have come out of it. It's a fascinating concept and an incredible way to use the power of the internet.

Adaptation is a necessary and powerful life process. But change is hard. It requires us to let go of many of the things that we *think* keep us grounded and safe. You need to find and utilize a lot of strength in this process, this we already know. But just as important here (and in life) is *flexibility*. Flexibility is something that so many of us struggle with, both physically and emotionally. When you allow yourself to bend and stretch with your journey, you are able to maintain a more powerful sense of drive, focus, and hope. It can feel strange to think and step outside of your comfort zone, to alter yourself, your actions, and even your beliefs. But this uncomfortable place is where most breakthroughs are made.

If you feel stuck, change something—anything. Keep moving. Keep flowing. Keep adapting. Stagnancy breeds turmoil. Flexibility cultivates life.

Afterthoughts + a Peek into the "Aftermath"

My ride through this process has been wild. It's been a journey of helplessness, frustration, realizations, healing, forgetting, and remembering. My "cure" ended up not being just one doctor, one diagnosis, one pill, or one dietary/lifestyle change. It was the accumulation of information, experience (of myself and of others), self-awareness, and perseverance over the span of more than six years.

It took that long for me to process everything, become shattered by it all, strip everything down, and begin to put the pieces of my health puzzle together in a way that could allow for me to save and live my life. It took focus, willpower, and dedication to my own life in order for me to power through the difficult moments, know that there was another side, and to believe that somehow I would find and experience it.

As I became more capable of navigating my way through the mess, I began to really learn about myself. I learned about what lights me up inside. I learned about some really poisonous emotional and physical habits that I had developed. I learned how to better process my emotions so they wouldn't become toxic sludge on my heart. I learned about the importance of self-care. I learned how to advocate for myself, not just in a medical context, but in *life*. I learned what it means to forgive everything that I cannot control. And most importantly, I learned how to really live.

After your life is threatened, you simply cannot go back to being the way you were. You have to change things. Because if you don't, you are ignoring one of the most powerful catalysts to your own health and happiness. The endless doctors' appointments, thousands of hours of online research, expensive tests and procedures, lack of social and emotional support—they can't all be in vain. They're meant to come together to shape how you can and will live in the aftermath of your illness. They are meant to make you better, stronger, and more alive than you would have ever been otherwise.

We all have a choice in life: We can either accept a victim mentality and feel sorry for ourselves, or we can let our terrible life moments empower us to become and do great things. This choice is not hard. Sure, it takes strength and a legitimate amount of work. But it's not hard to choose to live, even when things get really dark.

Looking back, there were so many times when I wanted to "be like everyone else". Not only did this fuel a ton of denial and ultimately, a lot of my illness itself, but it completely tortured me emotionally. It made me feel helpless and out of control. I was frustrated, confused, and I had no clue how to move forward. But the one thing that I did know was that I had all of the strength that I'd need inside of me.

Once I made a mindset shift and consciously decided to embrace my illness in a way that could be constructive, I committed to my path to good health with an intensity that I didn't even know I possessed. I became grateful for the different perspective on life that my illness had given me and promised that my experience would really mean something. I promised the universe that it would matter—not just to my own existence, but also to others' as well. I promised that with it, I would be and do great things.

Interest versus Commitment—Your Ultimate Call to Action

If you take one thing away from this book, I would like for it to be this:

How you choose to deal with your adversity (this illness) determines how it ends up affecting the big picture of your life.

I think that, generally speaking, most people are interested in living well. We are all interested in experiencing good health and feeling our best. But how many of us are really, truly committed to living this way? There is a huge difference between a genuine interest in something and a firm commitment to making that reality happen.

Ultimately, you are trying to survive. Survival is a basic human function that turns itself on when we are handed these "bad" cards. But survival needs to be about more than just staying afloat. It needs to be an intentional pursuit of *life*. It needs to be about doing your best in the here and now. Make lemonade, as they say. It's all about thriving in the thick of this adversity so that you can thrive on the other side of it too.

Get in Touch!

I would LOVE to answer any questions that you might have and connect with you regarding your own experience with an illness.

In other words, I'm here for you!

The best way to reach me is via email at:

bohannon.rochelle@gmail.com

Acknowledgements

I would like to personally thank *everyone* who stuck by me as I walked this crazy journey through illness and now health. There aren't enough words to express how grateful I am to have had your support and understanding during such a trying, chaotic time. You all know who are and I love each and every one of you fiercely.

Another huge THANK YOU to all of the doctors who served me with genuine compassion. I have kept your names private but you also know who you are. And, to every doctor out there who operates with a genuine love for their patients, know that you are a true gem!

I *need* to thank my husband, Brett, once more. Without his persistence, this book might never have made its way into the world. His enthusiasm for all that I do is amazing and I am so grateful to have such a supportive person to do life with.

Lastly, Self-Publishing School is gold! This program gave me the tools necessary to take action on this book and get it out there without the overwhelm that might have otherwise stopped me.

About the Author

A natural optimist and fierce independent, Rochelle Bohannon has been a lover of life since birth.

After battling and conquering a six-year mystery illness, she set out to have a real impact in the lives of others who have shared in a similar experience.

Ultimately, she is on a mission to empower others. Her illness was the catalyst and her desire to live big is the driving force behind this heartfelt duty to use her experience for something amazing. Thanks to the gift of adversity, she now wakes up each morning with a zest for life and a drive to *be* more and *give* more each day.

Her inspiring and holistic approach to living is what gives her an edge in life's big picture. Gratitude is her best friend, the sun gives her energy and love is what motivates her to live in a beautiful state of mind, no matter what.

Born and raised in southern California, with a grounding five-year stint in Portland, OR, Rochelle currently (and gratefully) resides in San Diego, CA with her husband, son, daughter and pup.

Thanks Again!

Thank you for reading *Stronger Than Sickness!*

If you enjoyed this book, would you take a minute to leave a review?

Simply head over to Amazon, search "Stronger Than Sickness" and leave your honest review.

Reviews help boost the visibility of this book so that I can get it into the hands of as many people as possible.

For more inspiration + life tips, visit me at thevibrantventure.com

Big love and vibrant health,

Rochelle